WHEN THE GYMS SHUT DOWN

LEARN HOW TO WORK OUT AT HOME AND GET YOUR
BODY FIT, TONED, AND STRONGER WITH
CALISTHENICS

YOUR FINE FETTLE

CONTENTS

Introduction   v

1. The Wonders of Working Out   1
2. Introducing Calisthenics   16
3. Eat Fit, Sleep Fit, Keep Fit   30
4. Set and Reach Your Goals   44
5. Home Fitness Perks and Pitfalls   57
6. Work Those Muscles   71
7. Managing Weak Spots and Injuries   86
8. Mega Movement Patterns   98
9. Over 30 Calisthenic Workouts to do at Home   111

Conclusion   129
References   133

A SPECIAL GIFT TO OUR READERS

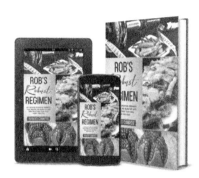

Included with your purchase of this book is a copy of Rob's Robust Regimen, to help you get started on your health and fitness journey and inspire you to create your own similar regimen to get where you want to be.

Click the link below and let us know which email address to deliver it to.

www.yourfinefettle.com

INTRODUCTION

We have all been there. Those broken New Year's resolutions, the promises to our doctor, or ourselves. This year I will drop the weight. This year I will get that six-pack. This year I will complete that marathon that has been on my bucket list for years. Okay, so the last one is a little extreme, but you have to start somewhere don't you? What is that old Chinese proverb? A journey of a thousand miles begins with a single step. You just need to start! So you do your research into getting a gym membership with a personal trainer. In your mind, you are planning which days you will be going to the gym and what exercises you want to try because you read that it would be great to help build your perfect body. But then you do the math and realize this is just not in your budget. Maybe if you drop the personal trainer you could afford it. Gym memberships can run anywhere in the region of about $700 per year (Crockett, 2019), excluding possible hidden costs such as sign up fees and surprise annual fees. You convince yourself that if you are going to spend this money you will stick to a daily routine of doing at least 30 minutes of some exercise. However, as time goes by you lose your drive or life simply gets in the way. Every day becomes a less and less occurring thing in your life and you go when you have time. By the end of the year, you realize that spending the money was a complete waste. What caused you to give up so easily? What excuses did you use? I was tired? I didn't have time?

Perhaps you didn't have the money to get a gym membership and you resorted to things like yo-yo diets to lose weight. Maybe you were able to stick to the diet for a few days, maybe a few weeks, before crashing back onto your previous habits and the weight coming back with a vengeance. Nothing fits. You are irritated and this leads to unhealthy coping mechanisms like stress snacking among others. No one likes to be overweight and it comes with many problems. According to the CDC (2020b), a person who is overweight can experience anything from depression, to sleep apnea, to death in very extreme cases. So in essence, carrying that little extra around the middle, thighs, or buttocks can have a serious impact on your health and well-being.

If the dangers are so well known why aren't more people trying to look after their health and weight? The answer lies in three important things: money, time, and taste. We live in a society that expects instant gratification with everything, be it food or even goals. We all have had days where you just cannot see yourself spending hours in front of the stove cooking or preparing a healthy meal when it is so much easier and faster just to get a burger or pizza. Junk food is convenient—plain and simple. Not only that, but it is cheaper than the healthy alternative (See, 2020). Plus, generally, it just tastes better. If you have a family that is living on a shoestring budget you go for the cheapest and easiest option to feed everyone. Now not all junk food is bad for you, moderation is of course key, but overeating and the convenience of this type of food do cause it to become an easy way out of cooking. However, you are slowly digging your own grave because of it.

These are the least of your concerns. You are so worried about getting fit, paying the bills, and putting food on the table that now you are losing sleep. A lack of sleep is just as bad as not getting exercise or eating unhealthy. The University of Arizona Health Sciences (2018) found that a loss of sleep causes cravings and even midnight snacking in people. Adding an extra meal to your day will cause your suggested calorie intake (2000-2500) to be exceeded. Exceeding calories only means one thing: increased weight, and sadly this is not muscle. Not only do you feel the need to reach for a snack when you can't sleep at night, but this can also affect you during the day. You need to function as a person when you are trying to do your job. Most people will turn to caffeine to keep them awake at work. The favorite is coffee, though tea and energy drinks do sometimes make an appearance, which can be drunk black or with milk and heaps of sugar. Sugar, the bane of everyone's existence. Between sugar and caffeine, you are bound to have another restless night.

It seems that everything is out to get in your way of that ideal body of yours. The gym is too expensive. Junk food is too readily available and tasty. Even losing a few hours of sleep a day can make you reach for that donut with your morning coffee. Losing weight now becomes a giant mountain to conquer that gets more and more difficult as the years roll by. Stop. Take a deep breath. Remember that single step. Start small. There is no need to get a gym membership when your body weight is the equipment you need and your home is the space in which you can train.

My body weight? But I am trying to lose it, how can it help me? Instead of bench pressing your way to those sculpted biceps, why not try Push-Ups or similar exercises? Guaranteed that will not cost you $700 a year. Calisthenics is the way forward when it comes to your personalized training program. Gone is the need for expensive equipment like bulky weight machines. The whole aim of calisthenics is that you use your weight to train your body into what you envision yourself being in the future. You do not even need to be an expert when it comes to doing any of the exercises. The exercises vary from beginner level, never even heard of calisthenics, all the way to expert level exercises that would amaze you. This type of exercise can target most muscle groups if you do the right exercise. You cannot train your biceps and expect a six-pack. Choosing the right exercise will yield the best results. What is important to remember when doing any form of exercise is that you are cleared to do exercise by your doctor. Always speak to your physician about any new exercises, diets, or changes to your life before implementing them, as they are the people who can give you the advice you need to start this journey.

What about cardio? Don't I need specialized equipment to get the cardio I need? Depending on the exercises you do you can easily raise your heart rate to those cardio levels. Burpees are a fine example of getting your heart pumping—just by hearing that word, as well as doing the exercise. Not a fan? Have a pair of sneakers? A run around the block or jogging on the spot are excellent ways to improve your cardio without the cost of a space-consuming treadmill.

I have old injuries, I shouldn't be exercising. That is an excuse. Unless a doctor has told you that you cannot exercise, then you can do calisthenics. Be the judge for yourself. With such a wide variety of different and unique exercises, you will find something that doesn't cause your injury to flare up.

I just don't have time! Another excuse. Do you watch television like a zombie? Why not try a few calisthenic exercises during your favorite show? An advert break? No problem, do five squats. Watching a movie? Every time a character does something that makes you laugh why not get up and do some lunges? It is easy.

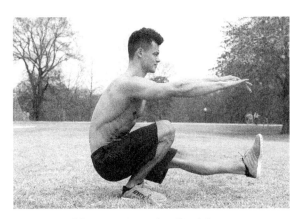

Man preparing to do a Pistol Squat.

Calisthenics is the way forward in personal home-training with little to no equipment needed. It doesn't matter if you are new to exercise or an old hand. Overweight, or skinny. Old, or young. There is an exercise for everything you can imagine BUT, you need to leave those excuses behind as you page through this book. Excuses only weigh you down and we want to throw that weight off, metaphorically and physically.

So, before you continue, please ensure that you have gone for your annual physical and discussed any new training programs with your doctor. Take this book along and show them what you are interested in trying. Remember, your health is made up of many parts and your doctor does play a vital part in it as well. Include them in this journey. You do not have to do this alone.

Exercise is always better, and more fun, when you have a partner who can encourage you, or you encourage them.

So, get changed into those shorts, a comfy top, and strap on your trainers. Keep a sweat towel close by and a bottle of water and let's get started!

THE WONDERS OF WORKING OUT

Exercise is good for you. No ifs, ands, or buts. However, exercise comes in many different forms, and often choosing the right one for you can be difficult, and this is where most people give up. The rest that quit are those that managed to find the exercise that they are interested in but the intensity or frequency of having to do the exercises is something they dread having to do. If you dread a workout maybe you need to consider a new workout, dropping back the intensity or number of days you train. That perfect body will not happen overnight. It takes dedication to get what you want. Start slow, start right, and keep at it.

THE BENEFITS OF BEING FIT

If there was no benefit to something you wouldn't likely attempt it. This statement holds no truer than when looking at why we should be fit. "Losing weight is hard. Being overweight is hard. You need to choose your hard." This anonymous quote holds very true to exercise. It is going to be an uphill battle but you need to start. It will be worth it. Whether you are trying to lose or gain weight or simply tone, there are massive benefits, both physical and mental, to be reaped from just attempting to get fit.

Physical Health

There are many benefits to your physical health (Robertson, 2017) when you start to exercise, no matter how small. One of the biggest benefits is not only the weight loss, if you are consistent in your training, but also keeping that weight off. Been struggling at work with getting your projects completed on time? Look no further than getting some exercise in. It has been proved to help with boosting productivity and reduce stress by controlling the cortisol in your body. Even problems like high blood pressure can be combated with regular exercise. If you are someone who likes the occasional jog this also has a great benefit in the fact that you are improving your cardiovascular health (Muscle Fit Pro, 2019). Heart disease is one of the leading causes of death in America, one out of four deaths is related to some form of heart disease, be it a heart attack or coronary artery disease (CDC, 2020a). By using excess energy on your training you will find that even your sleep will improve greatly. You will also find that if you are dedicated to your training you will start to make better choices when it comes to the fuel you put into your body. Once you are eating better and training well any digestion problems you had in the past will start to alleviate. Now that you are eating better and getting your body moving you are adding years to your life while fighting chronic diseases like diabetes and cholesterol. With consistent training, you will find that your muscles and bones are also improving in strength and endurance. This is where your nutrition plays a crucial role as your bones need that calcium as you are training. Thinking of adding on to your family? Yes, exercise is great for improving sex and maintaining a healthy pregnancy. The whole family benefits.

Mental Health

It is not only the physical part of your body that benefits from exercise but also your mental part (Robertson, 2017). As you exercise your brain is getting increased blood flow and it releases various hormones, such as dopamine and serotonin, which aids in improving your mood. A lot of people often don't want to exercise but once they force themselves to, then afterward they feel great, although a little tired. There is an old saying: if you look good, you feel good, and it is so true. Consistent training yields excellent results in your body and that boosts your self-esteem. Nothing better than getting those compliments and making yourself feel good about your new body.

EXERCISE IS FOR EVERYONE

Before you start with various excuses as to why you still cannot exercise, remember that exercise is for everyone. Unless you have been booked off by a medical professional, you can do exercise, irrespective of your age, weight, or gender. You just need to find the right exercise for you that gives you the best benefits. That said, the types of exercise that you should do is dependent on your age and fitness level.

Fitness for Young and Old

Physical activities that people are capable of doing can vary greatly depending on the age of the person. Let's divide the age groups up as early childhood (under five years of age), children and teenagers (5-18), adults (19-64), and senior adults (65+). Though not exercise per se, children under the age of five require light activity and some more energetic activity (NHS, 2019a). Depending on the age of the child, this could mean anything from simply rolling over to spending up to 180 minutes of playing throughout the day with activities such as skipping, running, or climbing. As they get older, children need different things from their physical activities. As they get more sure of their bodies, aerobic and strengthening exercises are something parents need to consider. At this stage, the children and teenagers should be aiming for about 60 minutes of moderate-intensity activity (NHS, 2019b) like walking, skating, or cycling. Moderate exercise means that there is an increase in heart rate, breathing, and body temperature. When strengthening muscles for the younger of the group, running is a great way to achieve muscle growth and endurance, and even team sports like basketball can help with this. For the older in the group, they can do more extreme sports like rock climbing to help with steady muscle growth.

Adults (19-64) should be getting a mix of moderate aerobic, vigorous, and very vigorous activity (NHS, 2019c), as well as muscle strengthening exercises, spread throughout the week. Be wary of just jumping into vigorous activity after a stint of no activity, you will cause injuries to yourself. Determining the difference between the various activities can be measured through your heart rate, either by your favorite fitness tracker or by doing some simple math. With moderate exercise, your heart rate should be about 70 percent of your maximum heart rate while vigorous exercise should raise your heart rate to between 70-85 percent of maximum (Mayo Clinic, 2019a). Very vigorous exercise can push your heart rate even higher than that but this sort of exercise should only be done for very short bursts, followed by rest, before continuing, and is known as High-Intensity Interval Training (HIIT) (NHS. 2019c). Examples of moderate exercise are walking or mowing the lawn. Vigorous exercise can include anything from swimming to jogging, or if you like speed, running. If you like the idea of

HIIT workouts, some of the best can be found by joining a spinning class. As for strengthening muscles, anything from carrying shopping bags or the kids will add the strength and endurance of your arm muscles, while gardening can work the other muscle groups such as your back or legs. Aim for about 150 minutes of moderate exercise a week or about 75 minutes of vigorous. Adding two days a week to work on strengthening your muscles is also a great addition to your training regime.

For people over 65 years of age, you can do the same exercises as those that are younger than you (NHS 2019d) if you have been doing these kinds of exercises before you reached this age. If not think of starting with light activities, such as cleaning the house before moving onto moderate and then finally vigorous exercises. Balance problems that can cause falling are easily rectified by doing exercises like yoga to strengthen the various muscles to prevent falls.

Age isn't a factor when it comes to doing exercise but rather just what kind of exercise you can do. So before jumping into training and ruining your drive or injuring yourself look at what you can do before attempting it. There is no shame in taking a step back before ramping it up to the levels you want to achieve.

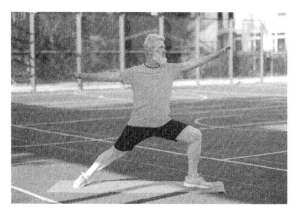

Man stretching with some yoga poses.

Male and Female Essentials

Are men and women so different when it comes to training? Naturally! It comes down to our body shapes and hormones (8fit Team, n.d.). Men tend to, but do not always, have a larger frame and thus more muscles, plus testosterone, as well as a larger heart and lungs to compensate for moving blood and oxygen to the various parts of the body. When compared to their male counterparts, females tend to be smaller in size but not necessarily petite. Ladies have estrogen and this tends to cause their bodies to hold onto fat more readily than that of their male counterparts. This is not all doom and gloom because they are more supple when it comes to exercises like yoga due to their more elastic-like muscles and they recover quicker after strenuous exercise. So does this mean men are just destined to bulk while women will remain flexible? No, not at all. Though most women like to turn to cardio machines to get their exercise and then stretching out with yoga and men like to "pump iron," this doesn't mean that the types of exercises are limited to gender. There is always a benefit to women, who have smaller, weaker, skeletal structures, to take the time in building their muscle strength and endurance by making use of weights or including weights in other exercises, like Squats or Lunges. Similarly for men, if they want to improve their flexibility they will need to concentrate on exercises that give them that bonus. So yes, our bodies make us different but it shouldn't pigeonhole us to certain types of exercises.

Another difference between men and women is where we get the energy to complete our exercises. Food is a valuable source of fuel but not all food is exactly what your body needs. Women tend to make use of fat reserves to fuel heavy sessions of training while men's bodies call for more carbohydrates in a combination with protein and some fat. This is why diets are vital when it comes to exercise.

At the end of the day, irrespective of your gender, you can achieve your weight goals with a combination of different training methods and a good, fueling diet.

WORKOUTS AT THE GYM

Exercise is great and all, but the motivation to do it is so hard to come by. This is where going to a brick and mortar gym can have so many benefits for you. The first is to get you out of the house—a change of scenery is always a great thing. You can argue that you could go to a park to get your run or jog in, or simply enjoy the sunshine while you do yoga and you'd be right, weather permitting. Good weather days do not stay all year round and eventually, the elements will turn on you (Schroeder, 2020). Very few people want to run in the rain and snow. Being able to go to a gym avoids stopping your training or giving it up completely. The gym can even be a social gathering area with various training classes offered by trainers in the gym. You can meet up with friends or even make friends while you are there. Training is a lot easier if you have a buddy system where you can encourage each other to get those training sessions done.

Many gyms have professional trainers, hired by the company, who are geared to help you with any of your fitness goals (Andy, 2018). These are people who specialize in making sure you are doing the exercises correctly to prevent injury. They are also very good at reminding you of your paid-for sessions and can be rather strict when enforcing exercise. Exactly what some people need in their lives. Some gyms even have great extras like pools, saunas, or even tanning beds (James, n.d.). At the end of the day, the gym is a great place to hide out if you need a breather from a hectic work schedule or family life, and let's face it, the membership is cheaper than buying the equipment your-self. Which brings us to the gym circuit. Anyone who has ever gone to a gym will know that there are a series of exercise machines, normally arranged in a circle, with a timer close by which forces you to move on to the next piece of equipment after a certain amount of time. Sometimes there is a stair-like structure in the center you will need to use between each of the pieces of equipment, to help with cardio. This is known as a circuit. This is a wonderful training routine that makes use of your whole body and brings cardio in as you run up and down the stairs, if available. As many parts of your body are being targeted, you can get multiple benefits, from cardio improvement to muscle endurance (Trainfitness, 2008).

STUCK AT HOME

A gym is a great place overall and it can be fun to get away from your busy schedule to enjoy some exercise but, what if we lost the gyms? The year 2020 has been a year of absolute turmoil. With the spread of the Corona Virus (Covid-19) worldwide, many countries closed not only their borders but also forced many people into lockdown. Effectively making us all prisoners in our own homes. In some places people were only allowed to leave their homes for food supplies or if they were emergency workers. Places like parks and gyms, a luxury that we often take for granted, were closed to the public in an attempt to flatten the curve of infections. This had disastrous effects on many people for several reasons, one of which was that they were not able to get the exercise they needed.

Now there were amazing people such as the athletes in Wuhan that managed to train in their apartments and Elisha Nochomovitz (Associated Press, 2020). You might be asking yourself who is Elisha Nochomovitz? If you don't know who he is by his name you may know him as the man that managed to run a marathon (~ 26 miles) along his tiny balcony (~ 23 feet). An amazing feat for an athlete but practically unattainable to someone who has not had the physical or even mental training to be able to complete this momentous task.

With lockdown came a variety of problems to our health. Firstly, depression was rising due to various reasons beyond our control (Aragona *et al.*, 2020), there was also an increase in alcohol abuse and even physical abuse. This not only affected adults but also children (Ramchandani, 2020) who suffered from anxiety as well as depression. With no way to alleviate the stress of the pandemic and depression, people seemed to be heading into a downward spiral. However, being trapped at home isn't all terrible. People can take the time to reevaluate their lives, bond with each other, and learn new skills. Earlier we read that exercise can improve our mood and even help with depression. Let's take a lesson from the Wuhan athletes and Elisha Nochomovitz: to exercise in small spaces is possible and would do you a world of good.

Look around yourself. Do you have a couch? One or two stairs? All of these items can be used in some form of home-based exercise. If you are particularly lucky to have a garden you can even use that to do interval running to help raise that heart rate to burn away calories of non-movement. As great as gyms are, we have learned that they will not always be there for us, so home-based exercises are the way to go to keep ourselves motivated to exercise. No more "I don't feel like getting in the car to drive to the gym" moments; you are home and you can train there. It just takes a change in mindset to encourage yourself to do it.

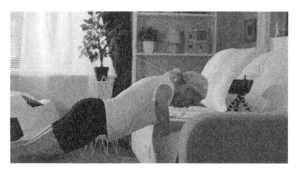

Anything can be used when you train at home, even the couch you normally relax on.

HOME-BASED EXERCISES

Depending on the size of your house, you may or may not have access to various types of training equipment, such as the stationary bike, treadmill, or even a weight set or two. For those of you that have smaller living areas, maybe even just a room which you share, you can make use of equipment like a jumping rope or resistance bands that come in varying resistances that suit your needs. The International Diabetes Federation (2020) makes some fantastic suggestions when it comes to doing home workouts. From three 20-minute sets (or an hour if you can) of brisk walking pace on a treadmill where you can also control the incline to get the maximum effort from the workout, to suggesting the use of bodyweight training such as Push-Up, Sit-Ups, as well as Squats and Lunges, which are the go-to for training leg muscles. If you are not big on cardio or strengthening exercises, try yoga to improve your muscles' elasticity and your flexibility.

There are pros and cons to training at home. There are a lot fewer germs as you are cleaning up after yourself at home. It doesn't take you forever to start your exercise as you are not waiting to get onto your favored equipment, there is no driving to a location involved, and it is by far cheaper to work out at home (Times of India, 2020). However, when you are at home you are not always as motivated as you would be at the gym, among other people that are also training hard. The variety of equipment at the gym will always be more than what you can have at home, plus they can afford to get new pieces every year —can you? Lastly, imagine you see an exercise that you believe is perfect for what you want in your routine but there is no one to teach you how to do it correctly, and this can lead to serious injury. Gyms have personal trainers who would be able to help you. Consider the pros and cons carefully before deciding to shell out top dollar for the equipment you may not even really need and do your homework about exercises, ask for help or turn to tutorials which you can find everywhere on the internet.

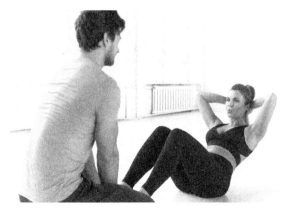

Get a workout partner to help out with your training regime.

NO EQUIPMENT NEEDED

To maintain a healthy body you do not need to spend a fortune. Generally, everything you need to get a full-body workout is all around you. Your body is the weight needed and an area a little bigger than an average yoga mat is all the space you need to get a decent workout in. Cardio is easily achieved with minimal space and a lot of effort. Very few things are needed for you to get an effective workout at home. It comes down to what you want from your exercise. Depending on the exercise, the equipment may change or not be needed at all. Doing Lunges or Squats requires nothing but your legs, but if you want to start doing things like Chin-Ups and you don't have a tree, then you will need to have a pull bar installed in your house or similar equipment. It is strongly advised that before you just go out and buy anything, no matter how cheap, you continue to read through the information in this book and look at the exercises suggested. Once you have decided on a routine then consider if you even need to invest in anything. You will be surprised that most exercises don't need any equipment. This is great because when the Covid-19 pandemic hit, just like toilet paper, most food items, and water, you couldn't find any free weights or home gym equipment in any of the major stores. If you were lucky to find anything of that nature you were shelling out top-dollar as everything was now overpriced.

So on that note, let's learn more about calisthenics and how our bodies can help us lose weight.

2

INTRODUCING CALISTHENICS

Maybe you have heard of calisthenics before but you have no idea where it is from. Though the origin of the word calisthenics is argued, what we do know is that it derives from the Greek words kallos (beauty) and sthenos (strength). The word was first used by Herodotus, a Greek historian, who used it to describe the training being done by the Spartan armies. This type of training was seen throughout the world in places such as Asia, India, and even Gaules just to name a few (Higgins, 2020). Modern-day calisthenics comes from Germany in the nineteenth century with the works from Friedrich Ludwig Jahn and Adolf Spiess who were trying to popularize the sport of gymnastics (The Editors of Encyclopaedia Britannica, 2020). Author Catherine Beecher, who was the first United States person to advocate for calisthenics, wrote a book called *Physiology and Calisthenics for Schools* *and Families* in 1857. And though it was primarily promoted to women, the exercise has now become popular with both genders. The health benefit of these sorts of exercises was noted at the beginning of the twentieth century and now is used in schools and even in the military to help with exercise and training.

WHAT IS CALISTHENICS?

Calisthenics is a type of free body exercise with different kinds of intensities depending on what is required by the practitioner. The range of exercises can include but is not limited to swinging, kicking, twisting, etc., and it is used to promote the body's flexibility, strength, and endurance and can even help with coordination (The Editors of Encyclopaedia Britannica, 2020). The whole idea behind it is to use your body weight as the resistance in your training instead of equipment like weight machines (Mazzo, 2019). It is quite literally the kind of training that can be done anywhere and at any time—you just need to be appropriately dressed. With calisthenics, the whole world becomes your gym. However, as with all things, there are pros and cons, and calisthenics is not excluded from this.

The first pro is that this is a very inexpensive type of training (Suarez, n.d.) with very little if any start-up cost needed. It comes down to what kind of resistance you want from your training. If it is too easy training with just your bodyweight you can consider resistance bands, which are fairly inexpensive and can be bought in many different resistance levels. Any place can be your gymnasium, be it at home, the park, or even when waiting for your kids to finish their after-school activities. As you need nothing but your body, you can train ANYWHERE! Calisthenics allows for functional fitness which is the kind of fitness you need to function as a human without getting injuries and maintaining a healthy body. It also helps with conditioning your body to achieve all your goals. Think of any movie you watched where people are training. Are they on a treadmill? Are they pumping iron in the gym? No! They are gathered on training grounds doing Jumping-Jacks, Push-Ups, etc.—all of that is calisthenics.

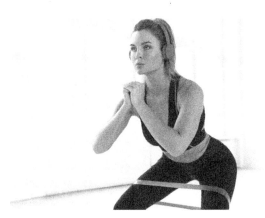

Add a resistance band to help you get an extra difficult training session.

As you get more experience in training in calisthenics you can start doing some amazing feats like Push-Ups while doing a handstand, which looks pretty cool. It also promotes not only strength but also stability, flexibility, and balance (Porter, 2020).

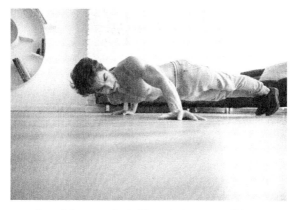

One of the many Push-Up variations you will learn with calisthenics.

Sadly, this is no miracle exercise and there are a few cons. Namely that it cannot be used as a form of physiotherapy (Suarez, n.d.). Calisthenics requires multiple muscle groups to work together to yield results. If even one muscle is not functioning the way it should, the other muscles overcompensate and the training will not yield the results that you want. Physical therapy after an injury or even surgery should always be done initially under the watchful eye of a therapist with controlled movements or weights. Don't get frustrated, this is all a process. Do your therapy, heal, and come back stronger than ever. Healing is part of the process.

Progression can also be difficult to see in the long run as there is nothing to gauge yourself against. In the gym you could be running those extra miles or lifting those extra weights, but when you do calisthenics you can't see that so easily. Your body weight is likely not to go up during this training as you are aiming to lose weight or tone. If you want more resistance, other than your body weight, you can consider using resistance bands or even weighted items such as weights that can be worn around the ankles or wrists, or even a weighted vest if you are really up to the challenge. This, however, does raise the cost of training.

Targeting a specific muscle group can also be quite hard to do when working on a routine but not impossible. Nothing says you can't bring weights into your routine if you want to build a specific muscle group (Porter, 2020). The same for cardio, if you are a person who loves watching the miles disappear as you run you will not get the same cardio and endurance training from calisthenics, which mostly concentrates on strength. Again, nothing stops you from incorporating a run into your routine if you want to work on your cardio. If you are the kind of person that loves the idea of large leg muscles, you will not get that from this type of training. Remember that you only have your weight to work with. You cannot bulk your muscles in your legs unless you add more resistance. You will have stronger legs but you will not get the bulk that you often see in bodybuilders. Lastly, even some of the simplest exercises can be challenging. Most people can't do a proper Push-Up with the right form, and that's okay. Start basic, do that Push-Up from your knees, and build it up to a full Push-Up. Most people find starting calis-

thenics too tough and will usually give up. However, it is important to remember that you need to start somewhere; build your
strength until you can do Chin-Ups with no assistance. It takes
time and dedication.

BENEFITS OF CALISTHENICS

By now you should be asking yourself, do the pros outweigh the
cons when looking at the benefits of calisthenics? With calisthenics, you can build some serious strength in your whole body
(Mazzo, 2019). You are not using some trifling weights, but
your entire body weight to do the exercises. You get better
movement from your body as this is functional training that
enhances the way you perform your daily tasks. Imagine being
able to carry four shopping bags from the car to your house
instead of just two. When training in calisthenics you are doing
compound movements and it requires all parts of your body to
work together to achieve what you want. You are meant to
work the whole body and not just part of it (Pearse, n.d.).

Another benefit is you have a better form (Mazzo, 2019). When
only training one set of muscles, people tend to pack on the
weights which can cause injury or other muscle groups to take
over the work and then you are no longer training the muscles
you wanted to train. With calisthenics, you can grow your base
strength before moving onto strengthening the various spots
you are interested in. When training you are concentrating on
multiple muscle groups rather than just one or two. You get a

better workout for your whole body instead of a percentage of it.

Calisthenics is great for your body as it can be gentler on your joints than most other exercises because you are working with your body's natural movements. The muscles develop along with those natural movements and your muscular structure and thus not putting any excessive strain on your body and reducing injuries. You also develop a good brain-body connection as you are developing your fine motor skills to help with all the actions you are performing. These movements are not all that easy to do as you need to be able to make split-second decisions to go with the increased flexibility, strength, and stamina of training.

You feel absolutely amazing! When you are 100 percent in control of everything you do you feel powerful. There is no greater feeling than knowing you are capable of doing anything you want. Do you want those perfect abs? Look no further than calisthenics. Activating and using your core is literally at the core of this exercise. Correct posture is key in training your abs (Pearse, n.d.). Remember, if your core muscles are strong your body is strong.

You can get a high calorie-burning workout from calisthenics. When combining short rests between sets you are burning through excess calories much quicker than other exercises that have a longer resting period. In a standard 30-minute training session, you can burn between 135-200 calories if your weight is between 125-200 lbs (WebMD, 2019); you will burn more calories the heavier you are, but not for long as you lose the weight. Calorie usage can be increased if you change the intensity of the workout. You can burn between 240-355 calories with a high-intensity workout, whether through shorter resting periods, or changing the body position when doing certain exercises. An example of this is the simple Push-Up. To make this exercise more difficult and increase the calories burned you can place your feet on a step (or two if you are brave) and continue the action.

With calisthenics, you can combine cardio and strength building in an all-encompassing workout (Pearse, n.d.). Combine your strengthening exercises with shorter rest periods, pushing your heart rate into the cardio range. As with all exercises, there is an aspect of discipline. This is the same with calisthenics, it isn't just about getting the exercise in and raising that heart rate, you need to have the discipline to be able to do those exercises and make the sacrifices to your time and even your diet. These exercises take time to learn and if you are not disciplined enough to put the time in you will fail.

You will never get bored with calisthenics. You do not need to limit yourself to just doing these exercises but can also combine it with weight training as well as cycling or jogging and running. Remember, the world is your gym, nothing stops you from doing a few Squats, Push-Ups, or other exercises during those sessions to get the maximum out of your training session.

This type of exercise is also great for weight loss (William, 2020) as it can increase your resting metabolic rate. This is where you burn calories while resting and is dependent on your muscle mass. If you have a large muscle mass you will be burning more calories than someone who has less. This is not the only way calisthenics can help you lose that excess weight. Strength training exercises cause your body to burn more calories after your exercise has been completed. So even if cardio burns more calories during exercise when compared to strength training, strength training causes your body to continue burning calories well after the exercise session has ended whereas, a cardio workout does not.

Lastly, calisthenics has something for everyone (Lyda, n.d.). Finding a regular Push-Up too easy? Change it to Diamond Push-Ups or Decline Push-Ups. Even an assisted Chin-Up could eventually become a One-Handed Chin-Up with enough dedication and training. You can be as creative as you want but be careful in not setting the bar too high for yourself. Everything takes time to learn and it takes a while to master calisthenics.

Calisthenics ticks all the right boxes when it comes to a unique, fun, and practical form of exercise. It can be done anywhere with next to no start-up costs and caters to the newest of the new and old hands when it comes to exercise. It has something for everyone and it definitely is a better option than trying to lose weight through extreme training or other measures.

THE SIX MAIN TYPES OF CALISTHENIC WORKOUTS

When looking at the human body there are six major muscle groups (Legge, n.d.) and they can be divided into the chest, back, arms, shoulders, legs, and calves. Knowing which muscles we want to work with can help us prioritize our training sessions. With calisthenics, six basic movements can be done to cover all the main muscle groups (Maximum Potential Calisthenics, n.d.). These movement patterns target muscle groups used for pulling and pushing, movements can be done horizontally or vertically, muscle groups used for Squats, and then the muscle chains found laterally (sides), anteriorly (front), or posteriorly (back), which can also be targeted with movements that can be done horizontally or vertically. Natural movements we do everyday target these muscle groups. Movements like squatting, bending over, pushing or pulling things, twisting, and lunging (Live Well Team, 2019) and it is with using these movements that calisthenics can target all the major muscle groups. By knowing which movements cause which muscles to activate, we are able to see that the various calisthenic exercises can be divided up into six distinct types of workouts.

The first of these workouts is called upper-body pushing (Robles & Robles, 2020), and this is where you concentrate on using the muscles of your upper body which includes the muscles in the chest, both the lateral and anterior of the shoulders, and triceps. The importance of exercising this part of your body is so that you can keep a stable position in your shoulders when pushing things away from you. Examples of exercises for this movement are natural Push-Ups, either against the ground or a wall.

The next movement is the upper body pulling which allows you to bring things closer to yourself. The muscles that are activated during these kinds of movements are the posterior of your shoulders, rhomboids, trapezius, latissimus dorsi (lats), and the biceps. Working on the strength of these muscles gives you the ability to be able to pull yourself up, either from the ground or if you are climbing over something. Chin-Ups or simply pulling yourself over a fence are examples of where you use the upper body pulling movement.

Next is the knee flexion (bending) movements which allow you to train the muscles which allow you to bend down and pick things up off of the ground. The muscles involved with this movement are exclusively in your legs—quadriceps, adductors, and glutes—while there are a few more muscles in your hips as well. Squatting is something that comes quite naturally to us as people but these exercises ensure that they are done correctly to prevent injury.

Then there are the single-leg movements that allow for improved balance when working with either one of your legs. The quadriceps and adductors also work hard when doing these movements but they are not alone. As the balance from having two legs is taken away your core muscles play a much larger role along with other smaller stabilizing muscles that would normally be at rest when you are doing exercises with both legs. The exercises are there to target your balance and coordination and could fix imbalances between the two legs that have accrued due to injury or surgery. Great exercises for this movement include Single-Leg Squats and Lunges. Remember that the exercises are for both your left and right leg, one set of these kinds of exercises is only completed when it has been done for both legs.

The hip extension movement targets the hamstrings, glutes, and the lower back, all in the posterior chain of muscles, which help with the flex and extension at the hip. The exercises for this movement aim to ensure that you are bending your hips correctly and preventing lower back injuries. Hip Bridging and Deadlifts are great ways to activate these muscles.

Lastly, there is the core stabilizing movements and this targets all the muscle groups of your abdomen, depending on what exercise you want to concentrate on. If your core is strong then the rest of you is strong. The best way to train your core is to Plank, regular or side, correctly.

To get a training session that covers all the major muscle groups combine, several exercises that target all the above movements over a 30-60 minute period, depending on your fitness. Choose your favorites or concentrate on certain muscle groups to get the best result from your training.

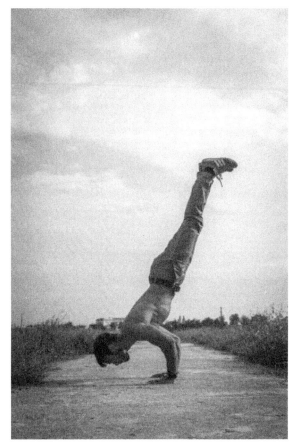

Man performing a Handstand Push-Up.

A lot of the calisthenic workouts look amazing, and often grav-ity-defying, so it is very important to remember that this is a level-based, beginner, intermediate and finally, expert exercise regime. If you cannot do a normal Plank you are not going to be able to do an Arm Extended Plank. Start with the easily achiev-able movements and exercises before training up to the more challenging ones by concentrating on your form while doing the exercises. It is better to do five perfect Push-Ups than 20 shoddy ones that don't do anything other than frustrate you and make you hate the process, or worse, injuring yourself and putting your process back by weeks, if not months. Nothing in life is easy, and if you want to invest in your health, then you need to realize that everything takes time. Dedicate yourself to the right form by spending the time perfecting it over days if not weeks. It isn't a race against anyone but yourself towards what you perceive as perfection. The more complex of the exercises build on what you do in the beginning stages, so, if you can't do the basics then forget attempting a Handstand Push-Up. Start slow, build up your base strength and form, then dazzle the world with your amazing calisthenics skills.

3

EAT FIT, SLEEP FIT, KEEP FIT

How many times have you seen an advertisement for some new training program or diet tips? All of which state that they will make you better, fitter, slimmer, or whatever catchphrase they used to get your attention. How many of those exercises and diets failed? It's likely a high number, and why do you think that is? Simple. You looked at your health as being dictated by either exercise OR diet. This is incorrect. In order to achieve the best health results, you need to consider not only diet AND exercise but also your sleep. An indication that sleep plays a crucial role in your health is when you are doing the exercise every day and eating well but you still feel exhausted (Sleep Foundation, 2019). The only thing you haven't incorporated into your healthy lifestyle was checking if you were getting a healthy amount of sleep.

Sleep, diet, and exercise are all pieces of a healthy lifestyle, miss even one part and you will never have a completely healthy life, and it can become a vicious cycle of repetition that will damage your body and give rise to serious conditions such as sleep apnea or even diabetes.

Choosing the right time to train is vital to your sleep health as training too late in the day—the usual benefits you get from training, raised metabolism and feeling energized—can now have a negative impact. Being more alert or having a higher temperature will cause you to toss and turn long after you decided to go to sleep. Although late afternoon training is great, as it is after work, try to complete your training session three hours before going to bed to allow for yourself to be calm when you snuggle into your sheets.

What you eat and drink can also have an impact on your sleeping habits. One too many late nights working or studying can cause you to load up on caffeine and sugary treats to try and remain awake during the day. This seems fine if you can manage to get through your day to get home but when you try to fall asleep you will note that caffeine especially affects your ability to fall asleep.

Lack of sleep is damaging in the short run and devastating in the long (Kittaneh, 2015). Losing but a few hours for a short period of time can cause your mood to sour, lower your judgment, and affect your ability to retain anything. Losing sleep over an extended period can cause obesity, diabetes, and early death. So think twice before cutting your hours of sleep. But then again, what is adequate sleep? This is where it gets a little tricky because it really does depend on you and what you feel is enough. Most people say that eight hours is the way to go but some people survive quite well on less than that—as low as five hours (Rampton, 2016). It all comes down to your internal clock (Bender, 2017). When we fall asleep, when we get hungry, and what we are able to do with our energy to remain active is all regulated by an internal clock, no two are the same so you must figure out what works for you. Take the time to get to know your own body.

FOOD AND FITNESS

Good foods versus bad foods—let's get this stigma out of the way early. What is good food? What is bad food? Can you even answer that? Vegetarians don't eat meat—does that make meat bad for someone who wants to eat meat? Sugar is bad for you. So I can't have my favorite fruit? There is no such thing as good food or bad food (Aimee, n.d.). Our bodies use all the food we eat as fuel to get through the day, whether that is some chocolate or a green salad; both are seen as fuel. The idea of good food and bad food can actually cause people to have issues with food and can lead to eating disorders. Moderation is key. You want that chocolate, have some. Do you want a green salad for lunch? Enjoy! A variety of food will give you the nutrition you need to be healthy. Having too much of anything will cause problems.

Most people like to speak about too much fat or too much sugar, but did you know that drinking too much water can kill you? So, in the future, when you think of foods, don't characterize them as good or bad but rather just think of them as fuel for your body. Some fuel gives your body better results than others, so consider carefully what you put in your tank. Don't always go for taste but think to yourself about the nutritional value and what your body needs. And yes, fat and sugar both play a role in a healthy diet, as long as you are not having too much.

Lifestyle and Nutrition

Food is important in our lives and the nutritional value of that food is what makes us function. You are what you eat, which holds very true when choosing the right diet. When you eat incorrectly it results in a body type that you may not like at all. One of the highest causes of poor nutrition is processed food. The reason we have processed food is that it lowers spoilage in food—it has better storage capabilities and is convenient. Grabbing a snack like a bag of chips off a shelf is so much easier than going home and preparing something.

However, there needs to be a trade-off for that convenience and sadly it is the nutritional content (Soud, 2014). During the production of processed foods, many vitamins and minerals are lost while there is an increase in additives and preservatives. Due to the preservatives, these meals tend to be very high in sugar and sodium and can contain allergies (please read labels).

Often there is very little fiber in processed foods and even ready-made meals—fiber is vital as that is the component in our meals that causes us to feel fuller longer and prevents us from overeating. Although these convenient foods are cheaper at the buying price they are more expensive for our health.

If you are not sure about what is processed here is a list of things you should probably avoid having too much of in the future:

- High-fructose corn syrup
- Trans fatty acids
- Artificial sweeteners
- Additives like sodium nitrate or monosodium glutamate (MSG)

Remember, you can still eat your favorite snack that may contain what is on the list but it should be done in moderation to prevent future problems. Eating too many foods that are processed can cause your liver to get sluggish (Commonwealth Sports Club, 2015) which causes your digestion to slow down. When your digestion slows down nutrients are not absorbed the way they should be. No nutrients means that you get no energy and with no energy, you become fatigued, and thus you cannot go about your normal day, much less try to exercise. If processed foods are your main source of fuel you are looking to a life of heart problems and diabetes.

Foods that are considered better for you are whole or natural foods. There is very little if any processing involved in these foods so they retain all their nutrients and vitamins. Nutrient-dense food generally has lower calories when compared to their processed counterparts. Fresh food items like meat, fruits and vegetables, and whole grains are natural food. Fresh foods, unlike some processed foods, break down completely and give us all the nutrients we need to maintain healthy energy levels throughout the day, plus the fiber makes your stomach feel fuller for longer. Whole grains are wonderful to your diet and it is strongly suggested if you don't have an allergy to add a variety to your diet. Whole grains cause your digestion process to absorb more nutrients by giving your digestion process time to break down the food completely. The fiber from these grains regulates your blood sugar as the conversion of starches into glucose is slowed. There are also phytochemicals, more so in whole grains than in fruit or vegetables, that are able to break down any carcinogenic chemicals. Fresh meat, when cooked correctly, contains beneficial fats—yes, some fats are better for you than others and your body needs them. Again, everything in moderation. Eating too much of a healthy thing can become an unhealthy thing.

Food isn't just about what is healthier versus what is not healthy; there are many other benefits to fueling your body when it comes to wanting something specific from your diet, be it helping with a cold you just can't shake or helping to lower the pounds that are sneaking into your waistline. Fruits like kiwis, red bell peppers, papaya, and any citrus fruit are great for the vitamin C boost (Healthline, 2020) you need if you feel a cold coming on as they are great anti-inflammatory foods. Vegetables like garlic, broccoli, and spinach contain vitamins A, C, and E as well as fiber and antioxidants. Spices like ginger and turmeric have long been known for the healing properties and have been used for anything from nausea to helping with rheumatoid arthritis and osteoarthritis. Seeds and nuts also play a vital role as sunflower seeds and almonds contain healthy fats as well as vitamin E and minerals like phosphorus and magnesium. Let's not forget dairy and meat. Plain yogurt, with no added sugars, is great as it contains live cultures that are excellent bacteria and vital for your gut health. Poultry is a great source of vitamin B-6 which keeps our red blood cells healthy, which is likely why we feel better after having some chicken soup. Making your own stock is easy and likely contains fewer processed items than the store-bought variety. For those that are not allergic, shellfish contain zinc which is vital to our overall health as this mineral is what keeps our immune cells functioning well. As for drinks, look no further than green tea (or tea in general); with a lot of antioxidants it is sure to boost your immune system. Along with moderation, variety is key. Loading up on just one of these food types will not make you healthy. Try several combinations to get the best results.

When trying to lose weight you need to look at your calorie intake. The average recommended calorie intake for a woman should be about 2000 while for a man it should be about 2500, all depending on the age, weight, type of lifestyle, activity, and overall health (Brazier, 2018). Before you drastically start cutting calories please realize that without calories we are unable to function. They are our energy sources. No energy means you cannot do anything. To lose weight safely, a deficit 0f between 500 and 1000 calories a day is needed to lose between 1 and 2 pounds a week (Bowerman, n.d.). However, if you cut back too much on the calories, taking in less than 1200 calories a day, you will not reach your body's requirements for nutrition. Rather combine the deficit of calories with increasing your activity through exercise. You still get to enjoy your food plus you are training your body.

So, we have looked at what is healthier to eat and how much we should eat but what about what is best for us when we become more active? Surely our food types should change to allow for maximum benefit? You are right. What you put into your body is what you get out of it. When choosing foods to complement your training look at consuming a variety of complex carbohy-drates (Zelman, n.d.), whole wheat bread, pasta, high fiber vegetables, and fruit, etc., lean protein, such as nuts, eggs, meat, etc., and low-fat dairy options. If you are someone who likes training in the morning, don't do it on an empty stomach, try some yogurt with low-fat granola. Prefer training in the after-noon and not hungry? Try meal replacement bars but check the label to know what is in it and the calorie amount. Eating well after your training session is as important as staying hydrated. Choose brown rice with some steamed veggies and grilled chicken. Feeling a little hungry during your main meals? Snacking is not bad; it is what you snack on that determines what is better or worse for you. Celery sticks or apple slices with some peanut butter and raisins are a great snack that gives plenty of fiber and energy that will carry you to the next meal. At the end of the day, you need to listen to your body and decide what goes into it. Think of the nutritional value and how much of it is processed and if that food type has a place in your life. No one can stop you from having that chocolate cake if you want it, remember, moderation is key.

Training alone cannot change our bodies. We need the right fuel to keep our bodies going and this is no different when trying to prepare ourselves for our calisthenics journey. Many of you must be cringing and thinking, "Oh here comes another diet plan I can't follow." Hold on, don't put this book down yet. This diet is surprisingly easy but will need a little self-control and time on your part to be able to stick to it.

First things first, and probably the toughest for all of us. Say goodbye to all your processed foods and empty calories (King, 2019). This means no more sweets, baked treats, all sugary or soft drinks, white bread, and rice. So, if it comes in a box or can, read the label. The second tough part, limiting the hours that you eat with intermittent fasting. Try to only eat for eight hours of your day. Less time to eat means you start looking at foods that make you feel fuller for longer. There is no need for intense calorie counting but try to stick to the calorie totals discussed earlier. Keep in mind you can still drink your favorite tea or coffee outside of the eating window if you eliminate sugar and milk (please don't dehydrate yourself).

That is the hardest part of this diet! So what can you eat? Whole foods will be your go-to for all your meals. Whole grains, fresh fruit and vegetables, lean protein, and various nuts and seeds. Plan your meals around whole foods and when you are feeling a little nibbly reach for those fruits and vegetables which are nutrient-dense and high in fiber. Worried about some of your foods being processed but still want to enjoy them, i.e., peanut butter? There are countless recipes online to help you make your own whole-food versions of your favorite snacks. Don't be scared to experiment.

Depending on what you want out of your diet and new training regime you may consider some form of supplements to help you. Supplements that can help with muscle growth and recovery include creatine and branched-chain amino acids (BCAA) while multivitamins are a good supplement for vitamins and minerals which help boost your immune system and keep you healthy. If you are someone who is prone to getting muscle cramps also consider looking into various electrolyte replacers and hydrate appropriately. You should speak to a medical professional before drastically changing your diet or taking supplements.

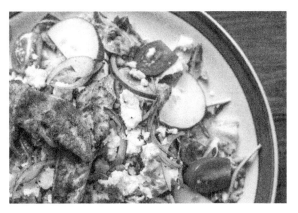

Grilled chicken salad, a perfectly balanced meal.

POWER OF SLEEP

Sleep is a wonderful thing. We need sleep as a species as without it there are many repercussions. But why does our body need sleep? During the day you are using food as fuel to keep yourself going but as night approaches you start to feel drained and exhausted and you just have to get some shut-eye (Chicago Tribune, 2018). Sleep almost seems like punishment for all the hard work you put into the day but you couldn't be more wrong. Sleep is possibly the most beneficial time of our lives. This is when your body can restore hormones that were depleted during the day as well as repairing anything that may need it. If you have ever had any kind of surgery you will know how important proper sleep is to your recovery period. Sleep promotes healing through the production of hormones and white blood cells while your immune system has a chance to fight any invading bacteria or viruses. Without rest, the immune system doesn't get a chance to recover and this is why you tend to get sick when you have not had any good rest.

Your body needs a break from your daily toils. The heart needs to slow down to recover, and blood pressure lowers with the hormones produced by sleep. These hormones also control your breathing by slowing it and all your muscles start to relax. Inflammation that had occurred during the day will start to heal. Your day was spent burning through calories to get the energy required to function but once you sleep this slows down considerably and your body gets to replenish the stock of stored energy, making ready for the following day's activities. Sleep is what determines the hormones that are released to make you feel full or hungry during the day. These hormones can be at the wrong levels if you do not get enough rest which can lead to under or overeating.

The physical aspects of your body aren't the only part of you that is affected by your sleep. Your mood is directly affected by the quality of sleep you get. When you are sleeping your body can concentrate on everything that needs to be fixed. The longer you remain awake the more strain you put on your body and the less time it has to recover from the day. Anyone who has lost a few precious hours of rest will be able to tell you how they "woke up on the wrong side of the bed" that morning. A common saying, for a common problem. A good night's rest means your hormone levels are replenished, your energy tanks are full, and your stress levels are very low. A bad night means the opposite.

Sleep Problems and How They Can be Fixed

Sleeping problems are very common. One such problem is insomnia, where people cannot fall asleep or even stay asleep, but this is only one of many types of sleep disorders (Mayo Clinic, 2019b). Sleep apnea prevents you from getting rest because of abnormal breathing. Restless legs syndrome (RLS) causes you to move your legs for no reason which keeps you awake. Then there is narcolepsy which lets you sleep but it is during the day and you tend to have no control over when and where you fall asleep. Other noteworthy disorders include parasomnia (sleepwalking) and sleep paralysis, which can be terrifying when you wake but your muscles are still paralyzed from sleep (ResMed, n.d.). Sleep disorders are terrible but they can and must be treated, whether with medication or therapy.

The most well known natural treatments to aid in sleep are melanin and lavender (Petre, 2020), and foodstuffs (Huizen, 2019) such as milk and even almonds (which contain melanin) can also aid you in catching those Zs you so desperately need. If you are allergic to nuts or milk, don't worry, making use of chamomile tea or even barley grass powder can aid your sleep. These are items you can quite easily add to your daily diet.

Food isn't the only thing that can influence your sleep. Your habits do as well. Avoid caffeine and alcohol before bed (Suni,

2020). Make sure your bedroom is only used for resting. Remove that TV or computer from the room you are meant to be getting rest in. Spend about 30 minutes before bed detoxing from bright screens such as computers, cellphones, tablets, etc., and pick up a good book to help you wind down before sleep. Sometimes sleep just doesn't come for a variety of reasons; if you are not asleep within 20 minutes, get up and go do something, in low light, until you feel tired, then try to go back to bed. Light plays a vital role in making us fall asleep and waking us. Having darker curtains prevents external lights from accidentally waking us or keeping us from falling asleep. A comfortable room and bed are also important so make sure that your room is at a pleasant temperature and the linen is comfy. Be strict with bedtimes to make sure that you get adequate sleep. If you know you are going to be getting up earlier, go to bed earlier! If sleeping problems persist for weeks on end you will need to go see a doctor.

At the end of the day, when you are well rested you have the energy to do what you want. Everything plays a role in your health. If you want the energy to work out you need to eat and sleep well.

4

SET AND REACH YOUR GOALS

We all have goals, but how many of us actually bother to think about the steps needed to reach that goal? We always seem to have that final picture in mind and we tend to forget that a lot of work needs to be done before reaching that goal. However, you have started. That's right, the very first thing you need to consider is your goal. What do you want to achieve? I want to lose weight! That's nice, how much? In what time frame? Are you going to weight train? Cardio? Diet? There is so much that needs to be considered before just jumping in with both feet, which is likely why so many people fail in their weight loss journey. They have a goal but no plan.

THE DIFFICULT QUESTIONS

Yup, we are starting here, trying to answer some questions about ourselves we would rather not.

- What do you want?
- How will you achieve it?
- What is your motivation?
- What is your training strategy?

If you cannot answer these questions do not start a new diet or exercise regime because it will fail. You need a plan and you need to stick to it. By answering these questions you will be able to put a fully functional plan into action; if you are being realistic, it is one you will be able to achieve.

This brings us to the next important point: research. You need to do the research about your goals. Want to lose weight? Look at what your options are. Look at what you are capable of. What should you eat? What are you willing to give up: time, money, or your favorite treats? There is no easy way out—if someone tells you there is, they are likely trying to make money out of you. Research everything and decide for yourself which strategy is best for you. If you do the work you are likely to see it through to the end. Get yourself a fitness journal—any old notebook will do—and keep notes of everything you are planning, step for step. There is nothing better than being able to tick something off once it has been achieved.

The reason you chose this book already shows that you are in the right mindset for change. You have been equipped with the knowledge about food and sleep, and now it comes down to what you want to gain from calisthenics. What do you want from this exercise?

Focused Exercises

After you have set a goal for yourself the next step is to think about what types of exercises will get you closer to that goal. Exercises can be divided into four main categories: strength, balance, stretching (flexibility), and cardio (aerobic or endurance) (Harvard Health Publishing, 2019). Exercises that target strength are the ones where weight is being used, and it aims to build your strength. Strengthening your muscles also aids in bone growth, lowers blood sugar, and helps with weight loss. Muscles that are strengthened correctly also help with posture and can improve balance. Good posture and balance prevents injuries in training or just living your everyday life. Having great balance prevents falls and makes you feel steadier on your own feet, or foot, depending on the training you are doing. Exercises that are great for balance include tai-chi, yoga, and many exercises in calisthenics, namely One-Handed Push-Ups or even a Handstand. Even if you feel your balance is perfect it is never too late or too early to start working on your balance and making improvements.

You cannot forget the health of your heart and lungs! All cardio exercises work on your endurance and the health of a vital set of organs. Anything that causes your heart to beat faster and makes you take deeper breaths is termed as cardio workouts. Doing endurance training is great for your body in other regards as it lowers body fat and blood sugar levels, and it just makes you feel good afterward. Then there is flexibility. You may not think much of flexibility but as we age it gets significantly more difficult to touch our toes, much less try some of the crazier yoga poses. Muscles and tendons tend to lose their elasticity over time and to prevent atrophy it's a good idea to do some stretches. Be careful when you do your stretches as the muscles need to be warm before starting a stretching routine. Try a short walk of five minutes before you start.

With the range of move sets in calisthenics, everything mentioned above falls into it quite well. Some moves are easier to perform while others require you to have the basic moves in a perfect form before even attempting the tougher move sets. Once you know what it is you want from your training you are able to choose the types of move sets you want to concentrate on. It sounds easier than what it looks like because before you choose what you want to do you need to be honest with yourself as to what your capabilities are. Start small and build up to where you want to be, don't start at the top, it will only cause frustration and then failure.

Going for the Prize

In order to build a house, you need to have a solid foundation. This is true for everything in life. Do you want that CEO position? You need to put the time in for your studies and then work hard. Calisthenics is no different. Not everyone can do a Handstand. Not everyone can do a Push-Up without resting on their knees. People are different. Do not compare yourself to someone who has been doing this for years (Jackson, n.d.-a). It is one of the worst things you can do and can cause you to lose sight of your own goals. A journey has to start somewhere and if it is a Push-Up from your knees then you are still one step ahead of anyone else who hasn't started.

Calisthenics is a great way to have fun and experiment with what you can and can't do. If you are not enjoying your current exercise routine, scan the internet, this book, or ask someone at the gym for new routines you can try or new move sets you can work on. This is a rapidly evolving exercise and people are always coming up with new moves. However, if you are trying something new, make use of having a partner so that you can be assisted if something were to go awry. Boasting is something you can do in moderation. Be proud of your achievements, show the world what you can do.

Todd Kuslikis (n.d.-a), also known as Bodyweight Todd, shares similar thoughts with Jackson (n.d.-a) when it comes to starting with calisthenics. He goes on to elaborate on his insights about calisthenics which should help you with knowing where your abilities lie. Firstly there is your focus which can be divided into three parts: short, medium, and long. Basically, it comes down to what you want from your training today, within three months, and what is your overall goal. You need to be able to set goals for each of these phases of your training. Along with your focus, you need to decide what you are concentrating on in terms of your training. If you are trying too many things, then you are not really concentrating on your goals. Bring your focus together on a few basics and once they are mastered, move onto trying new things. Be consistent—no one ran a marathon by training haphazardly. You need to decide on your training days, how long you plan to train, and what you will train. Having good training habits is what will push you to achieve those goals. Every training session, focus on the now and give it your best shot! We all stumble and fall but it is those of us that get back up that show the true results. Your mindset is what pushes you through difficult days. Earlier we discussed the importance of sleep and eating well; these are non-training factors that can influence how well you are able to train. Recovery is vital to all forms of exercise, as that is what builds your strength and endurance. No recovery means no gain, so take the time to relax between training sessions.

Keep it fun! There is nothing as disheartening as losing interest in something you love. Keep it fresh, challenge yourself, or go back and refresh on your basics. Do whatever gets you to do those sessions every week. Luckily you are quite spoiled for choice with calisthenics. It is because of the different types of exercises that you need to not only put the hours into your workouts but also in your research. Each move set has its bene-fits and combining several can give you the best well-rounded session where not only all your muscles are targeted but you are also combining all the focused exercises. Don't flounder away in the dark not knowing what you are doing and possibly getting injured. Arm yourself with the knowledge to reach your goals. Then, be patient with yourself. What is that old saying? Rome wasn't built in a day? And neither will your perfect body. Training takes time, a lot of time. The more you train, the more time you take to perfect the basics, the better your outcome in the future. But you need to get through the boring stuff first, and sometimes it is tougher than what it seems to be.

However, sometimes our patience is lost completely and we want to give up, and you know what? That is okay. Know your limits, know when you need to step back and say to yourself "I can't do this." But, didn't you just speak about not giving up on your goals? True, but you do not need to give up on your goal. Maybe a move set is too difficult. Maybe you had a bad night and you got no sleep. Maybe you even skipped a meal because you were too busy during the day. All of this can affect your mindset when you are in the gym trying to train. Rather give up on a training session one day than giving up on everything and saying, "That's it! I'm done. I quit!" One day is one day, take the time to recover and come back tomorrow to try again. Maybe even re-evaluate your goal. Perhaps it is too difficult. Look at achieving small goals in between that are more obtainable.

Lastly, learning all the skills required to master calisthenics ends up becoming a habit. You have spent time learning the basics and all the advanced skills are built from knowing the basics. In the future, there will be more exciting and vastly more difficult move sets so if you treat your learning as a habit you will continue to not only grow as a person but you will obtain those goals you want to achieve.

Setting goals is the foundation to exercise. What do you want? Do you want to run a mile in under 10 minutes? Do you want to attempt an L-sit for 10 seconds or longer? Both seem momentous tasks but they are equally achievable if you have the right goals in place to help you. Jackson (n.d.-b) puts it rather elegantly. A goal is but a dream unless you take the time to write it down. "Nonsense! If I have a goal in mind that should be enough!" It isn't. Goals need to be seen daily. This reminds you of what you are working toward. Take the time to write it down and put it in a place, or several places, where you can see it every single day. When you have that bad training session or you just can't be bothered to do a training session, look at it and remind yourself why you started this journey in the first place.

Now we get into the nitty-gritty part of goals. They need to be specific in their nature. You are likely to stick to a goal that is specific rather than general. Before setting that goal think of asking yourself five questions. Why am I doing this? Express the purpose of or the benefits of this goal to you. What do I want to accomplish with this goal? Weight loss? Toning?

General fitness? You need to be sure of this. Where can I go to achieve this goal? Do I need access to a gym or can it be done from home? When am I able to work on this goal? Knowing when you can get the best out of your training is vital to keeping yourself going. Some people need coffee to get out of bed, some need a good work out session. For calisthenics you could even ask which are the best work sets to get the best results from? There are so many questions you need to be able to answer before being sure of your goal. Go through all of them.

Your goals need to be measurable, otherwise, how will you know you are getting anywhere in your training or if you have reached your goal? You can decide how to measure your goal, be it in pounds, inches, or the ability to do certain move sets. Goals need to be achievable. If a goal is too far above your reach then you will not obtain it. Work in smaller goals or time frames to achieve certain goals to help you reach that final goal, or you will end up being sorely disappointed in yourself. However, be realistic with your goals and timeframes. If something is too difficult it will be too frustrating to complete and if it is too easy there will be no challenge and no need for you to really apply yourself for it.

Do you have more than one goal that you would like to achieve? Just like the focus that was discussed earlier, goals need to be divided into different time-based levels: short, medium, and long-term. Setting yourself achievable goals while aiming for that big goal is the difference between maintaining the will to achieve it or giving up completely.

Once all of that is decided it is important to realize that reaching your goal is not as important as your health. With the repetitive nature of the movements in calisthenics, you are opening yourself up to potential injury if you overtrain. So don't go overboard with trying to reach your goal; all good things come with time. Consider your number of sets and the rest in between carefully before just jumping into something new. Listen to your body as well as your head.

That's another thing: your mindset. It is easy to think of a goal and it is easy to write it down but how easy is it to keep up the willpower? You cannot get your body into shape if your mind isn't ready to join it. You read about all these great training exercises and the fun people are having and you want to join in, but when you do you get nervous about what other people think of you or how you will look. So you avoid the gyms, you avoid the mirrors. Don't do that to yourself. Keep that final picture of you in your minds' eye. Start with smaller workouts, things you know you can do to achieve your short term goals. Don't get locked into a routine. If you want to get a quick run in before starting your calisthenics workout and the treadmills are all full, don't quit; even though the frustration is understood, choose something else to push your heart rate up. Variety is key so that you don't get bored. Switch up what you do to keep yourself motivated.

Accountability is something else you have to work on (Holland, n.d.). No one stops you from working out, especially at home. You need to make a conscious decision to skip working out and then you have no one to blame except yourself when you do not reach your goals in time. If you are training alone think of creative ways to entice yourself to go training. Keep your sneakers close to your written-out goal so that when you see them you are reminded of your goal. Or get a training buddy—there is nothing better than a person who has your back and can call you on your accountability if you want to skip training for no valid reason.

And yes, there will be bad days and bad training sessions where you feel like you want to throw the towel in but that is where a healthy mindset and your consistency come into play. It's one bad day—don't let it become a bad week by skipping your training sessions and pigging out on junk food. Nip that in the bud right now. One bad day doesn't have to be the end. Wrap up your training with something easier, go home and think about what may have caused it. Did you sleep well? Eat well? Once you have worked through it then try again tomorrow but never stop. The point of a bad day is to see if you can bounce back from them.

Reward systems are also very important and are completely dependent on who you are as a person. Rewards can range from paying yourself to train (Guerra, 2017), a couple of dollars an hour which can be used to buy yourself something nice when you reach a certain total. Some people prefer to cave to their sweet tooth after some training. Why not hit a certain number of training hours then reward yourself with something that you are craving—just remember your calorie deficit, so don't go overboard. Perhaps you prefer to reward yourself while you are training? Instead of being cooped up at home why not go to a park or the beach to get some training in? Fresh air and beautiful scenery is always something that makes most people happy. Or, do nothing. Seriously, do absolutely nothing for an hour or two after you are done training. Watch some television, read a book, or simply take a nap. Anything can be a reward for training if you want it to be.

Diarize Everything

So your goal is visible for you to always see but what about your achievements? Pounds do not always drop very quickly but inches do. Get yourself a diary to document everything. Take before and after pictures. Write down what you attempted in your training, sets, and repetitions in those sets. Discuss how you felt about the training session, positive and negative feelings. Write about your mood before and after the session. Documenting your fuel consumption would also be beneficial as you can directly see which foods affect your training. While training, moods, and fuels should be documented daily, it is not suggested that you measure yourself as frequently. There is nothing more disheartening than not seeing the physical results of your training. It takes time and if you are going to watch it that closely you are not going to see the fruits of your labor and you will likely stall or quit. Do an initial measurement before starting your goal then don't look at it again for at least a month. Even if the changes aren't noticeable they are there. Take it one day at a time.

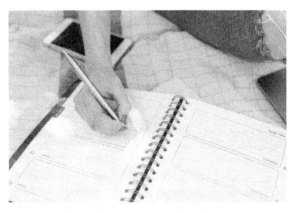

Remember to write everything down.

5

HOME FITNESS PERKS AND PITFALLS

.

If there is anything the lockdown during the Corona (Covid-19) pandemic has taught us it's that we can survive being forced to stay in our homes for extended periods of time. For some of us, it has been a positive experience with growth while for others it was filled with stress, doubt, and confusion. Though there were some positives for some people a lot who relied on going out and training were feeling the urge to do something, anything, to get their muscles fired up. And though running across balconies was one possible way to get exercise, not everyone had that luxury, however, many of us do have space within our dwellings that is ours and that is more than enough to train from home.

PERKS OF TRAINING FROM HOME

So why is training from home easier than packing a tog-bag and heading to the gym? There are a ton of benefits to be had. If you happen to be one of those people who now work remotely there is no traveling to be done on your part (Cronkleton, 2019a). Even if you don't work remotely you still have to go home at some point, so when you are home fill up that water bottle, get changed into training clothes then get started. Training from home is significantly cheaper than joining a gym with little if any start-up cost for any equipment you may need, as you will mostly be relying on your own bodyweight to train. Never again do you have to wait for the gym doors to open for early morning training. If you want to start training at 4 am, go for it. It is your home, you can do as you please. It is because of this that you no longer need to feel self-conscious, especially if you are new to training and may feel a little like an hour old foal that has no idea what to do. You have your own pace and there is no need to push yourself beyond this if you are not comfortable.

There is also no age limit when working out at home (Delavier & Gundill, 2012) which is great as calisthenics has no age restriction, but certain gyms don't allow anyone under the age of 16 through the doors. Gyms are a great place to be social with friends but sometimes this can be detrimental to your training especially if you are trying to concentrate on your workout and someone wants to chitchat. As you are training in a place that is yours, it stops the urge to show off in front of others and turns your training session into an ego-boosting session. There is nothing worse to your training regime than trying to top someone else; remember, you are doing this for you, not to make someone else feel inadequate. Once ego walks out the door you are able to concentrate on your goals. When home most distractions that you would face in the gym are eliminated, namely time limits on pieces of equipment or having to move from one place to another to allow others to use the equipment like weight machines. When you are in your own place you do not have to concern yourself with other unknown people, or germs (Guerra, 2019) which is an immediate boost to your immune system. Plus, when you are in your own home you can take your time perfecting the move sets from calisthenics without someone hovering over your shoulder waiting for you to complete your set so that they can sweep in and use the equipment after you.

Training from home forces you to use your brain as you need to start doing your own research and thinking of ways to do various exercises. You are forced to be creative (Kelly, 2016). Though, that said, you can no longer be that creative with your excuses to not get some training in. "I don't feel like it" is no longer going to cut it. You only need 30 minutes a day to get a beneficial amount of time for exercise.

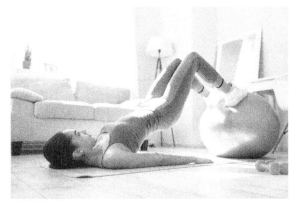

Your own space, your own time, and your own equipment.

So all in all, training from home has some very nice advantages. Time is money and you are saving a lot of it.

PITFALLS TO TRAINING AT HOME

Like so many good things in life, there is always something that has to be the opposite and sadly this is also true to training from home. With the convenience of training at home, some people think that you can now train every day (Coleman, n.d.), at the same intensity, with no break for recovery. This is the worst mindset to have. You are making your muscles stronger and in order for the muscles to get stronger, you need to allow them time to rest. Overtraining can result in injury and a lowered immune system, just to name a few problems. Incorrect weights, or levels of difficulty, can also have an impact on the gains you want. With calisthenics, you do not have to use weights but there are body positions that can make it more challenging to complete. You need to be able to choose the right style for you to get the best workout, otherwise it is too easy or too difficult. This will help with your resistance training. Cardio —you need it, whether you run or have less rest between sets. However, too much is worse than having none.

When people sit idly or when it is cold their intake of fluid tends to be lower than when they are active or when it is warm. Dehydration is one of the major pitfalls of training anywhere. If you do not consume adequate levels of water you will soon find yourself on the receiving end of cramping muscles. However, do not think of dehydration as a lack of water, this is only one part of it. When you sweat you are also losing vital electrolytes which are the reason our muscles can work (Yu-Yahiro, 1994). A lack of these electrolytes can wreak havoc on a body that is trying to train hard. If you are someone who finds it hard to consume liquid, not just coffee and tea, during the day try adding fruit or just plain lemon to your water bottle. It refreshes you and puts some of those electrolytes back into your body. During your training, you can also make use of various energy drinks, though you should have a look at the sugar content before deciding which you would use.

As people, we all have a comfort zone that we are not always willing to leave and this is where many people stop their training journey. You need to be able to challenge yourself so be wary of training sessions that are too boring or not challenging enough. Switch it up, change it around, make exercise fun again. For you to be able to do that you need to have a plan. This is why your goal needs to be written out. You need to do the research before just jumping into exercise.

If you are planning on using intermittent fasting be warned that your morning training will be affected by it. You can train on an empty stomach, a lot of people prefer it, but do not expect a lot of power if there is no fuel in the tank. Then there are your workout clothes. You may not think much of it but the right gear can mean the difference between a great workout or feeling like you can't get anywhere. Aim for something light-weight that can prevent you from sweating too much or hampering your movements.

Choosing the correct room to train in is as important as which clothes you wear or what exercises you do (Ellis, 2020). A room that has too many distractions, such as your bed, a TV, or a computer, can be your downfall. You need to be concentrating on your exercises and not needless distractions. Not all distractions are static, sometimes you may have kids that are underfoot and that is just as bad as considering a nap during your routine. Include the kids in your exercise, either they join in happily or they run for hills and leave you alone—a win-win situation really. Watch out for other potential dangers that are in a room before doing your exercises. No one likes banging their head on a window or pulling a table over onto themselves. A little common sense goes a long way when it comes to unnecessary injuries that could have been avoided just by taking the time to look for potential dangers. Repetition is bad, if you are doing the same training exercises every single day you will grow bored and unchallenged. The point is to improve, not stagnate. Switch it up with different types of move sets or difficulty levels to keep your body, and mind, entertained. Another mistake that is often seen in training from home is not concentrating on your form. The correct form is everything in calisthenics. It can be the difference between growing your strength correctly or a one way trip to a serious injury (Ling, 2020). Having someone to help you with the correct form or paying close attention to doing your basic move sets perfectly before moving on is crucial to your growth. Take things slow and do it right the first time.

Many people overlook two very important parts of their training as they are usually too excited to just jump into the training. Warm-up and stretching (Langley, 2020) is every bit as important as the actual training. If you do not do a warm-up routine before your main set of exercises you will damage muscles and if you do not stretch upon completion you risk the chance of muscles cramping or pulling tight which can affect your posture. Take the five minutes to warm up and the five minutes to stretch at the end. Your cup of coffee can wait till your entire routine has been completed.

The last two points are something that needs to be discussed for exercising as a whole. The first is not to believe everything you see or hear about exercising (Bode, 2003) on social media. What is advertised is not always true so make sure to read the fine print before buying into anything. With that said, it is vital for you to consult an expert, be that a doctor, a physiotherapist, or dietician, before making drastic changes to your training session or eating habits. They are the experts for a reason, not listening to them can have serious repercussions.

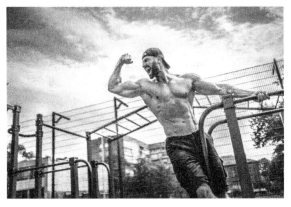

Don't let anything get in the way of what you want to achieve.

HAVE THE PERKS OUTWEIGH THE PITFALLS

There are a lot of pitfalls when it comes to training at home in comparison to the perks, however, most of the pitfalls have to do with your willingness to train while others are things you simply need to consider and change about your environment. Meaning that all of those pitfalls can be overcome with a little effort on your part. If you are unsure of what you want from your training session just remember the basics that need to be covered: warm-up, cardiovascular, resistance, flexibility, and cooling down. Once you have these basics you can concentrate on what you want to put into them. Be creative but do your research and stay within your capabilities.

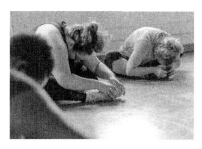

Women stretching after warm-up.

Warm-up:

Irrespective of what some people may think, warming up your muscles is singularly the most important part of your training (Cordier, 2018). In order for your muscles to function at their peak, they need to have oxygen readily available to them. To have this oxygen they need to be at a higher temperature than when they are resting. Your heart is not just an organ but a high modified muscle that also needs to be warmed up to function at its best. Warm muscles are less prone to injury as the elasticity improves, which means less painful cramps or possible muscle tears. These muscles are now ready for stretching. This time is also used to mentally prepare you for the work you are about to put into your exercise. You can concentrate on making sure the muscles you are going to use are sufficiently ready to be used, especially if you are going to be doing strength training. Warm-ups can be anything from jogging on the spot, light cycling, a walk, or doing one or two rounds of your strength move set at a much lower intensity.

Cardiovascular (Cardio)

Do you have a staircase in your house? Can you climb it without feeling winded? No? Then your cardiovascular fitness is not good. Arguably, after our brains, our hearts and lungs are the next important parts of our body. A strong cardiovascular system means your heart and lungs are able to deliver blood and oxygen to the various places in the body. Aerobics exercises are meant to strengthen your heart and it has so many benefits (Marcin, 2020). Having a healthy cardiovascular system means you can battle the bulge, asthma, high blood pressure, back pain (swimming); it also strengthens your immune system and improves your mood. Aerobic exercises are not just for the young, the elderly get lasting benefits such as helping with balancing problems and preventing falls. And let's face it, nothing makes you sleep better than 30-60 minutes of moderate to intense activity during the day. When people think of cardio training they immediately think of jogging or running but these are not your only options. Swimming is an excellent form of cardio training with little stress on the lower extremities. Walking and gardening are also great ways to get that heart pumping! If you cannot put a full cardio workout in then break it into 10-minute sessions during a day just to get your heart pumping. This is great with calisthenics as you have multiple repetitions of exercise sets with a little rest so it is guaranteed to push your heart into that perfect fat-burning range.

Resistance

When you ask people: Why do you do resistance training? The likely answer will be: To build muscles of course. This is only partially true. Resistance training is partially for building muscles but it is also to improve the strength of ligaments, tendons, and bones (Better Health, n.d.). Most experts recommend at least two days of strength training a week while resting muscle groups up to 48 hours before training them again. There are so many benefits to resistance (strength) training that can either be physical or mental. Strength training allows for calories to be burned well after the exercising has been completed so it helps to burn fat, tone, and strengthen muscles, improves stamina, mobility, posture, balance along with aiding sleep, self-confidence, and self-esteem. This is also great for the elderly as improved bone density and muscle strength can prevent falls, or if a fall happens, that bones do not break. To get the best from your strength training there are some principles that you must understand. What exercises are being done? What is the intensity of the workout? How many exercises are in the set? How many repetitions (reps) of the exercises are you going to do? What is your rest period between sets? And lastly, how often will you be doing these training sessions in a week? This is why your research is so important before jumping into any kind of exercise. Resistance training can be done with or without equipment. If you have access to free weights they are a great addition to any resistance training program. If not, don't fret, your own body weight is more than enough to get the right training out of your muscles. Exercises like Squats, Lunges, Deadlifts, Push-Ups, or Pull-Ups cover a wide array of muscle groups and you do not need equipment to handle them.

Flexibility

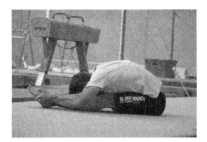

Man with extreme flexibility.

Now you don't need to contort yourself into a pretzel to be able to do calisthenics but some decent flexibility would do you a world of good. Why work on flexibility when you just want to lose weight or build muscles? Because you cannot do that if you are not flexible. When you are flexible you can have a wider range of movement (Cronkleton, 2020) as well as improved balance, which is exactly what you need with calisthenics. Flexibility can be difficult to achieve but the benefits are worth it. If your muscles can do what you expect of them you will find that your training yields fewer injuries, there is less pain after training, it can lead to greater strength which leads to better physical performance, and lastly, a positive outlook on your training. When you can do what you set out to do it is a great feeling! A good stretching session is wonderful. Think about when you get out of bed in the morning. One of the first things you do is stretch and take a deep breath, and with that, you are ready for the day. If you want to improve your flexibility look no further than yoga to help you out. Many of the stances in yoga aim to help with stretching muscles of various groups.

Cooldown

We have all been in a training group and you hear the instructor yelling that there is one more rep before you are done and they say to push yourself. You finish the rep and you want to collapse from fatigue and then you hear those dreaded words: Cooldown time! You are exhausted, why should you do a cooldown? Many people tend to leave a training group without completing a cooldown and it is one of the worst things you can do to yourself. There are benefits to doing a cooldown (Cronkleton, 2019b, Frey, 2020). It slows your breathing, heart rate, temperature, and blood pressure to return to what it was before you started exercising, or at least close to it. A steady cooldown allows for your blood flow to steadily slow down instead of dropping straight back to relaxed blood flow. This is very important, if the blood flow is not regulated properly excess blood is left pooled in your lower extremities' veins, and with the lowered heart rate it is difficult to pump that blood back to where it should be. This can lead to a person feeling dizzy, feeling sick, or even passing out. Stretching during this stage will also help with the reduction of lactic acid, which is what makes your muscles feel sore after a workout. And overall it helps you to relax after a long training session and since you put so much work into your training you deserve some time to just relax. Depending on what exercises you did will depend on what cooldown you should do. If you went running, walk for a cool down, or do standing quad stretches. Yoga is a great way to cool down and can stretch a wide range of muscles and allows for your heart rate too slow to a nice pace where you can feel you are no longer gasping for air.

So, sticking to those five basic factors of exercise will allow you to have a productive and satisfying training session, irrespective of what you are training in, be it calisthenics or training for a marathon.

6

WORK THOSE MUSCLES

E arlier we discussed the major muscle groups in a human body, that being the chest, back, arms, shoulder, legs, and calves. Each muscle set is composed of different muscles that are connected to various parts of our bodies. Some are stronger than others and that is why it is so important to train them right from the start so that you have a base strength to work off of. When considering your training there are three muscle-specific training structures you can follow. There is the full-body workout (Friedrich, 2019b), the split system training (Rogers, 2020), and then concentrating on a single muscle group (Friedrich, 2019a).

A full-body workout is as it says, you train all of the muscle groups during a singular training session. The muscles act as a singular unit instead of part of one and this causes the functionality of your body to be better, improving your daily life. One of the benefits of this kind of training session is something called proprioception. This is like a sixth sense where your body is able to read where it is in a certain space, i.e. you know exactly what your arms and legs are doing as well as their positions at any given time. You cannot over-train specific muscle groups when using this approach as the muscles are all being used at the same time. Doing a full-body workout does not require multiple training days but only a few as you are concentrating on all your muscle groups and they will need time to recover between each training session.

The full-body workout is not without its own drawbacks. The first of which is that it's not precise in the targeting of a partic-ular muscle group. Though great for a beginner, this structure is not that great when building strength. If your muscle groups are not of equal strength, then training with a full-body structure will never give the lagging groups a chance to catch up to the stronger muscle groups. A full-body workout is tiring and if you push yourself too hard, you are going to find personal growth is nay impossible or you may need more time to recover. If this is the case then it is suggested that you try the split system training instead.

The split system can be implemented in many ways but the most common seems to be dividing the body into the upper part, chest, back, and arms, and the lower part, legs, and the buttocks, while any core stabilizing exercises can be done within each of the groups. The benefits of this type of structure are that you are able to get more intense workouts in comparison to the number of days you have to rest from it. For example, if you train your upper body you need about 48 hours to recover properly before you can train it again, but within 24 hours you can concentrate on your lower half, thus getting two days of training in with the full-body workout you would only have had one. Being able to work the muscles a lot harder, you will be able to get better results from your training.

However, if you are someone who is just starting out or has a limited schedule this is likely not the kind of training schedule for you. Missing a training session means that you miss several muscle groups being trained which can lead to your progress being skewed against full-body development.

Though not ideal, training a specific muscle group does have an advantage. If a muscle group is underdeveloped or recovering from injury or surgery, then this is a great way for it to catch up to the other muscle groups. Sometimes when training with the full-body structure there are some muscle groups that do lag behind, so be mindful of this when you plan your training sessions so that you can keep an eye on your development and see where you need to compensate.

Sadly, with this structure, there are a lot of cons, namely the exercises used to target single muscle groups don't always mimic our natural movements, i.e. a bicep curl isn't used in our daily lives, unless it is to show some muscle; whereas bending over to pick something up uses our core, back, and arms. There is no cohesion between the other muscles in the same group and offers nothing to the overall functionality of our body. The next is that when training one group of muscles there isn't as much energy used as when training your whole body, so fewer calories are used.

At the end of the day, you are the one that needs to make the decision as to the manner of your training. It is suggested that you look at what your base strength is and then decide on what needs work where. If you find your arms are not strong enough then consider a split structure; however, if you are recovering from a sprained ankle work on that leg's strength until it is ready to join in a full-body workout. Trust in your capabilities, do your research, and do not be scared to talk to experts who can give you more advice.

MUSCLE-SPECIFIC EXERCISES

If you have ever spent time in a gym or watched training videos on Youtube you would have noticed there are literally thousands of different ways to get a workout. It can be confusing and annoying to find the right type of exercise that you want to use in your training and this is where most people decide to just give up. Don't do that. The different muscle groups are going to be the guide that is needed to choose the right exercise for you.

Chest Muscles

When looking at the anterior (front) part of the chest you will see the pectoral region, your pecs, which is made up of four different muscles, pectoralis major, pectoralis minor, serratus anterior, and subclavius (Jones, 2020a). These muscles help us to move the upper arm across the body (Legge, n.d.). Due to the different points that these various muscles are connected to our body, it allows for different movements. There are horizontal movements, where the arms are pushing from the front of the chest, which is used in bench pressing. This stimulates the sternocostal head of your pectoralis major which is the set of muscles that attaches your sternum to your rib cage. Then there are vertical movements, where the arms are moving upwards away from the chest, like when you do an incline bench press. With these exercises, you are stimulating the smaller part of the pectoral major called the clavicular head, which is the set of muscles that attached the collarbone to the upper arm. Exercises that work all your chest muscles, as well as some of your arm muscles, include a various number of bench presses. But if you want to concentrate on not using any equipment then you can use a large collection of different types of Push-Ups that are available to you (Robles & Robles, 2020) as well as Dips, which can be done with a sturdy chair or table or against a stair. Even ladies can have a well-defined chest that does not make them look like ripped bodybuilders. Lighter weights and bodyweight training allows for more definition and not to bulk. Try

Planking for a workout that will not only work out your chest muscles but also your arms and shoulders (Mercedes, 2019).

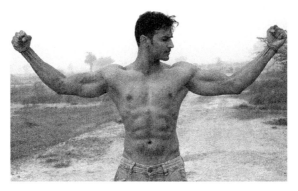

Well defined anterior muscles with no bulking.

Back Muscles

Your back isn't just one sheet of muscle but is made up of three main regions called the superficial, which controls the movements of the shoulder, intermediate, which controls the movements of the thorax, and deep back muscles, which have to do with the movements of the spine (Jones, 2020b). The muscles that you concentrate on when working on your back are the trapezius (also known as traps), rhomboids, latissimus dorsi (lats), and erector spinae (spinal erectors), with the first three being in the upper region of your back and the last being in your lower region running up along your spine (Legge, n.d.). The lats keep your upper arm attached to your back while the trapezius connects the shoulder blades to the spine with the rhomboids to help with the stabilizing of the shoulder blades with an extra connection to the spine. The spinal erectors do just that—they stabilize your back, which many people need as they sit too much.

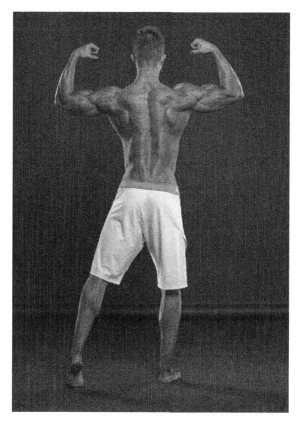

Well defined posterior muscles with no bulking.

Overtraining any one of these muscles can lead to back problems so it is a good idea to develop all four of these back muscles simultaneously to prevent problems. Deadlifts, Pull-Ups, and

Pull-Downs are the best workouts for your back muscles and they are all possible with or without going to the gym. With some equipment, like resistance bands, you can easily simulate a Lat Pull-Down. If you do not want to invest in any equipment you can simply try Supermans or Downward Dog Pose (Bhanot, 2017), which are great for your back and your abdomen. Most people try to hold their breath while doing this exercise, but you shouldn't. Starving your muscles of oxygen prevents them from doing their job.

Arm Muscles

We use our arms in every activity we do. Even when we sit at our computer we are working the muscles in our forearms as we type. Try reaching for your coffee and see the rest of your arm muscles start to work together. Your arms are divided into three parts: the upper, lower arm, and your hand, all of which have their own unique muscles that achieve the movement that is needed in daily life. When training, only four main muscles are concentrated on and these are the biceps brachii (also known as biceps), biceps brachialis, triceps, and the muscles of the forearms (Legge, n.d.). The biceps brachii is a muscle that has one connection close to the elbow while it has two connections up in the shoulder, while biceps brachialis is found under the biceps, and together these muscles are in charge of the flexing action of our arm. This is not the only thing this set of muscles can do. The twisting of your lower arm from palm down to palm up is also controlled by them. Triceps perform the opposite job to the biceps and push the lower arm away from the body and is made up of three parts (tri = three; bi = two). Forearm muscles handle the more intricate tasks of our daily lives, such as typing and writing and this can lead to underdevelopment if not trained correctly. Luckily these muscles tend to workout just as hard as their larger counterparts when the right exercises are chosen. As for the exercises associated with these sets of muscles, they tend to overlap with other exercises such as those that concentrate on the back or on the chest, which is great, more muscle groups getting trained at once. Any form of Curling (raising the lower arm toward the shoulder), Dips, Chin-Ups, and Pull-Ups are the way to go with working those arm muscles. Once more, these exercises can be done with or without equipment. If you are more partial to not having equipment why not try Planking, Push-Ups, or if you are very brave Burpees with a Push-Up (warning: advanced levels only!) (Tucker *et al.*, 2020).

Shoulder Muscles

The shoulder muscle is known as a deltoid and is made up of three parts: the anterior (front), lateral (side), and posterior (back) heads. The deltoid as a whole is a very important muscle as it is in charge of stabilizing various other muscles when they do their tasks (Legge, n.d.). When the lats and trapezius muscles work to bring your arms behind you, your rear deltoids are helping. The front deltoids aid the pectoral muscles to return your arms to the front of your body. When you raise your arms to your sides it is the lateral deltoids that help the trapezius, pectoral muscles, as well as those in your neck and back to achieve this task. Here, the angle at which you do your training will affect which part of the deltoids is being targeted. Aim to do exercises that target all regions to avoid over and underdevelopment. Bench Presses are a great way to work your anterior deltoids while Side Raises aim the work at your lateral deltoids. Bent-Over Rows aim to work those posterior deltoids. At home, you can make use of Push-Ups to work the front deltoids, Side Raises with a resistance band for the lateral deltoids, also, a Bent-Over Row while holding onto a resistance band as you are standing on it; it will be perfect for your rear deltoids. When using a resistance band be sure to know your capabilities, as normally the resistance bands are color-coded for different difficulties.

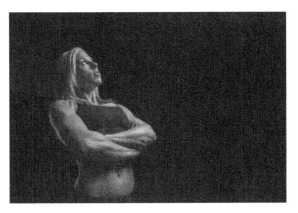

Well defined shoulder and forearms on a woman.

Leg Muscles

Let's divide the leg into two parts: upper and lower. The upper part of the leg consists of the major muscles for the quadriceps (quads) and is found at the anterior of the body, as well as the hamstrings and gluteus (glutes) which are found in the posterior of the leg (Legge, n.d.). The lower part of the leg is made up of the calf which will be discussed after this, as the exercises aimed at those muscles are significantly different from those aimed at these large muscles. As the muscle groups for the upper leg are so diverse they will be discussed separately as their exercise is also quite different depending on which muscle group you want to concentrate on.

When working with the quadriceps (quad = four), the large muscles to train are the

vastus lateralis, the vastus medialis, the vastus intermedius, and the rectus femoris. Together these muscles cause the downward hinge motion of the hip and the extension of the knee from a bent position, so those are the type of exercises that are used to train these muscles. Squats and Lunges in any form will help these muscles to reach the levels you want them to be at. If you want to increase the difficulty of your squats without adding weights try the Bulgarian Split Squat.

Next are the hamstrings which consist of three muscles on the back of your leg called the semitendinosus, the semimembranosus, and lastly the biceps femoris. The hamstrings do the opposite of the quads, they straighten the hips and bend the knee. The quads and glutes are sadly the main areas of focus for most people and the hamstrings sadly lack the training they need to help carry the body through exercise. Injured hamstrings are a common injury in sport (Higgins, 2019). This is due to two reasons: weakness, which can affect your posture and lead to back pain, and tightness, as a tight muscle can tear and lead you to have it corrected surgically. Squats are not a good option here as that concentrates more on the quads, rather try Deadlifts or Hamstring Curls to work those hamstrings. You can also give Inchworms a try. This is where you are in a plank position on your hands and you slowly inch your hands back a few feet then move forward again. Hard work sure, but so worth it.

Lastly, there are the gluteus muscles (your butt) which are made up of three muscles called the gluteus maximus, gluteus minimus, and the gluteus medius. The muscles are there for stabilizing all movements during your leg training sessions. If after a training session you find your rear a little sensitive when sitting, then you know you have targeted the right muscle groups for that perfect butt. All the exercises previously mentioned play a role in the development of these muscles but if you would like more of a challenge you can try Dumbbell Lunges that add an extra level of difficulty to your regular Lunges as there is more weight to be lifted. There are a ton of exercises you can do without any equipment at all. Walking

Lunges, Step-Ups, and even Bridges (Eisinger, 2017) all give that extra burn in the derrière.

A lot of the exercises are similar but it is a good idea to carefully look at what muscles are being targeted by what exercises so that you do not let some of the muscles get underdeveloped which could lead to injury. Careful research and planning are your best friends when it comes to getting the best out of a training session.

Calf Muscles

People often joke with bodybuilders and say that they skip leg days due to underdeveloped calf muscles, but the reality of the matter is that it can be quite difficult to get the results that you want from your calves due to limited training that targets them. Each calf is made up of two muscles: the gastrocnemius which is overlaid on the second muscle, called the soleus (Legge, n.d.). Exercises for the calves can be divided into pressing, pushing something away from the body, and raising, pushing the body away from something. Though the exercises lack a flare as with other exercises, it seems they can all be done with next to no training equipment unless you want to use weighted items. Standard heel raise from the floor is good enough, seated or standing, but if you want a bit more of a challenge try doing them from a stair and drop your heel below the level of the toes. Not difficult enough? Single-Leg Heel Raises are there to increase the challenge, and these can be done assisted or unassisted. When in doubt, grab hold of something and make sure your knee is not bent or you are getting those quads to help and that is not the point.

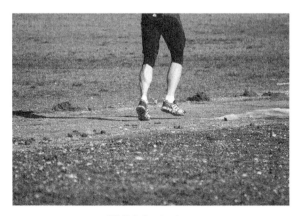

Well defined calves.

What about the core muscles? Is there nothing special to discuss with the core muscles in mind? Not really, no. Though many people are obsessed with getting the perfect abs, few exercises target them without targeting something else. When you are training the other muscle groups you need to engage your core and make it strong, but simply doing the exercises shown for the different muscle groups is enough to get your abs trained. Having a strong core is important because it does stabilize the spine and helps with the bending of the chest towards your feet.

Now that you have the know-how of what muscles are worked with what exercises you can start to consider how you want to break your training up during the week. If there is an underdeveloped muscle group you can take the time to concentrate on it. If you are more comfortable with a full-body workout you may have to have a longer session, up to an hour, but will need a longer recovery time. If you prefer the split system type of training, then it is easier with recovery between the different muscle groups, but if you skip a day of training you will find that one muscle group doesn't get the attention that was given to another. Sticking to your decision is what is important here.

7

MANAGING WEAK SPOTS AND INJURIES

You may have heard the phrase "No pain, no gain." Take that saying and throw it out! There is a difference between a muscle straining and one that is screaming for you to stop what you are doing. Pain is the body's way of telling you that something is wrong. Pushing through a warning from your body can be catastrophic and can result in torn muscles, broken bones, or worse. Know your capabilities and your body. Know when to push and when to let up, this can mean the difference between 'gaining' or losing.

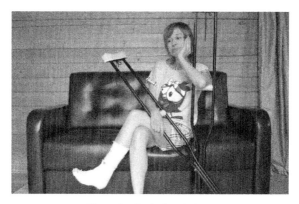

The sad setback of an injury.

PREVENTING INJURIES

Getting injured sucks, there is no way around it. It is costly, painful, and can result in months or even years' worth of training being thrown away. Some of the most common training injuries include sprains, strains, and joint problems (Harvard Health Publishing, 2013). Many injuries can be prevented by you being careful, knowing your capabilities, and making sure you are in a safe environment, whether that is at the gym or home. The first step to preventing any injuries is talking to your doctor. They are the ones that can make educated decisions about what your body can and can't do. They are a helpful resource of information and can easily put you on the right track for never or seldomly getting an injury. Listen to your doctor! This cannot be more overstated. Choose the correct workout for your level. Don't think that on your first day of training you can just do a Handstand Push-Up set. Know your capabilities. Start slow, everyone has to start somewhere and the beginner level eventually falls away to the higher levels.

Warm-ups are crucial—a cold muscle is one that can tear. Get the heart slowly pumping by doing a five-minute brisk walk and some stretches afterward to get the best benefit from your workout. Don't hold the stretches for too long either; 5-10 seconds is good enough. When doing the exercises you have decided to do, know the correct technique. A good technique means you are not only doing the exercises correctly but you are concentrating on the correct muscle groups and there is no compensation by other groups. Stay hydrated. You may not be a plant but you too can die if you do not drink water. Exercise is a sweaty business and you need to replace the lost fluids before you become dehydrated. Don't forget to make sure you are also replacing your electrolytes to avoid cramps. The correct gear for the correct exercise is also vital. Don't think walking shoes are good enough for a hard session of Lunges and Squats. There is nothing more distracting than aching feet when you are trying to exercise. To avoid injury due to repetitive exercises, vary what you do to get the maximum out of your workout. Know when to throw in the towel—overtraining is just as bad as no training. Don't forget to reset your body by cooling down for between 5-10 minutes. Your tired muscles will thank you tomorrow.

When you are training make use of progressions to prevent injury (Quinn, 2020). Progressions in strength training can be changed with increasing set, reps, or adding weight. By combining these factors you will easily be able to judge where you are in your training. If it is too easy add more sets or reps and if it is still too easy, increase the weight (or difficulty level). If it is too difficult then cut back. Knowing when to raise the level or drop it back is crucial to building a strong body and preventing injuries.

Don't discount a good massage after a tough gym session. You can do this yourself or have someone do it for you. Massages are great as they can reduce the pain (Conner, 2017) associated with training too hard, increasing the blood flow, as well as protecting and fixing problem areas plus who doesn't love a great massage? However, if there is a serious problem, i.e. pain that refuses to go away after several days or weeks it is a good idea to seek the assistance of your doctor or physiotherapist to see if there is an underlying problem.

Even if you are careful while training and you take all the precautions and you look after yourself, accidents do happen and you need to be prepared for them mentally. There are few things more disappointing than a major setback in your training. It can make or break a person when they are hit with an unexpected injury that requires a significant duration of recovery time. It can be tough but the first thing you need to do is accept the fact that you are sidelined, but know that it is only temporary (Dellitt, 2018). Choose what to do with the extra time you now have, don't get bored, do research, and see what you are able to do in terms of exercise in your current condition, after discussing it with your doctor. Keep up with whatever diet you have been following, don't let the depression of not training affect your eating habits. If you are able, depending on your injury, try some low-impact exercises to still keep you somewhat active.

There has been a slight setback in your training, that is alright, don't obsess about it, rather think of it as you hit the pause button until your recovery is complete then you can come back stronger than ever. Now that you have time to sit and research why not consider some new goals to help you prevent this injury in the future or consider ways to strengthen the area that has been injured. A positive mindset about an injury can mean the difference between overcoming or succumbing to it.

Common Calisthenic Injuries and Dealing With Them

As the pros and cons go hand in hand, so do risk and reward. Earlier, the reward of doing calisthenics was discussed and all in all, it sounded wonderful but no exercise is without its own risks. According to the National Electronic Injury Surveillance System between 2007 and 2016, there were nearly four million injuries that resulted from various gym equipment as well as calisthenic exercises (Verbanas-Rutgers, 2019). Those affected were mostly white men between the ages of 20 and 39 with injuries to the knees, ankles, and shoulders. Likely the causes of these injuries are due to people looking up the various exercises online and then trying to master them with no previous training or supervision. During this time even more serious injuries were coming to light such as nerve damage, puncture wounds (the reason for a safe environment to train in!), and even internal injuries. It is for this reason that it is so important to start with the basics, build up a base strength then advance with time. Jumping to the most advanced of the movements might look awesome but it will cost you. A study was done in 2018 by Kaiser *et al.* (2018) where a sample of 184 people was taken (156 men and 28 women) to ascertain the kind of injuries a person who trained in calisthenics would pick up during exercise. By the end of the study, it was noted that the most prevalent injuries were the tendon and muscle injuries (~ 44 percent and ~ 26 percent respectively) and these injuries were most found to have occurred in the shoulders as well as hands and wrists (~42 percent and 19 percent respectively). A total of 77 percent of people who reported an injury, 72 people who had 124 injuries, exhibited an upper-body injury. Some injuries were rather serious as there were dislocations as well as fractures.

Don't let the numbers fool you, they seem high but Kaiser et al. (2018) states that though the injuries are similar to what is seen in gymnastics the injury risk is actually lower. Irrespective of this, people who make use of this kind of training should be familiar with the risks and think about a sufficient prevention strategy to curb the risk of injury. Verbanas-Rutgers (2019) suggests that anyone who is using calisthenics to train other people should make sure that their clients are in the right condition, use the correct form, and make use of the recovery time to allow for proper rest between sessions.

Calisthenics is training where you are going to do a lot of repetitions of similar exercises in one training session and this can lead to repetitive strain injury (Cyborggainz, 2020). Because of this, it is very important to change your training and avoid working the same set of muscles too often. Recovery is vital for preventing injury or healing. Fall injuries are also something that is seen in calisthenics, i.e. trying to do a Single-Arm Pull-Up and not being quite ready for it yet. Prevention is always better than the cure so be mindful of what you do and where you do it.

So, we have been injured doing calisthenics, or falling down the stairs, what do we do? According to Thevendran (2017), most people don't care how they heal but rather when they will be healed and this is the wrong mindset to have. Recovery is essential to the overall health of a person and allows for healing of the injury so that the person can return to some normality if an injury isn't too severe. When an injury occurs that results in redness and swelling the first thing that must come to your mind is R.I.C.E.: Rest (get off the injury as soon as possible), Ice (cold therapy to help with pain), Compression (soft bandages wound around the injury to prevent too much swelling), and Elevation (raise the injury to prevent swelling due to gravity). Used mostly for soft tissue injuries this is a vital practice that will help reduce the swelling and to jump-start the healing process. Don't use the injured part of your body, splints and braces are a great way to prevent too much movement in the affected area. If you are particularly good at using bandages you will be able to bind the injury to prevent any movement. You cannot heal from an injury if you are still doing the movements that can aggravate the injury.

Injuries will hurt, there is no way around that but if it continues for longer than two weeks it is time to consult your doctor to see if further steps need to be taken. However, when an injury occurs you need to be mindful of how it feels. Is it a simple strain or is it something more serious? If you cannot walk like you normally do, if you are bleeding or the bones look misaligned, don't wait to see a specialist, go straight to the closest emergency room, and get yourself checked out (Testa, 2018).

Physiotherapy, if you are prescribed this please go do it! No ifs, ands, or buts. A physiotherapist is a person who will give you the treatment that is needed for you to get back on track to a normal life. They are also the ones you can ask about when you can return to training. They are likely to give you exercises to help with movements to accelerate healing. This will also help with muscle wasting away due to the non-movement rest. Don't forget your diet! Protein, vitamin C, and D, as well as Omega-3 fats help with muscle building, collagen production accumulating calcium in the bones, as well as limiting inflammation, and promotes a speedy recovery.

Importance of Progression and Regression

Calisthenics has a wide range of movements that you can try your hand at. Some are simple, such as a Wall or Inclined Push-Up but can increase in difficulty with different move sets, such as the Handstand Push-Up. In order to get to the most difficult of the move sets, you need to understand how the progression of any of the exercises is done. Being able to do movement patterns that build on a particular exercise you want to do is something that needs to start simple and move forward. What are movement patterns? These are patterns of movement we follow when we do anything, i.e. bending over, squatting, etc. Working on these patterns is what gives us the ability to work up the strength required to do more difficult calisthenics (Roam, 2015). Progression is measured in sets and reps, of which everything needs to be in a good form (Maximum Potential Calisthenics, n.d.). Only when you are able to do those sets and reps perfectly can you move onto the next progression in the movement set. Starting with the basics is what builds your base strength for the future. However, what if you cannot do the more difficult parts of the movement pattern? Then instead of progressing you regress the movement to one step earlier or straight back to the basics (Schifferle, 2015). If you cannot maintain the correct form when doing an exercise there is no point in continuing at that level—drop back and try again, or take a cool down and come back after some rest. Continuing to do the exercise incorrectly can result in the wrong muscle set from working or incurring an injury.

Know Your Weak Spots

Before you start any kind of training program you should be asking yourself: can I do this? Am I capable of starting and finishing this? Not everyone is equal. Different genders, different body sizes, and different histories all play a role in whether you will be able to handle calisthenics. The first thing you need to do is identify if you have any weak spots (Jackson, 2016a). What can't you do? You need to be honest with yourself as this is a way to prevent injury. Once you know what your weaknesses are you can work on them to make them stronger or to just bring them up to the level that is required to start the base strength training for calisthenics.

If you have chronic pain with or without exercise it is a good idea for you to have a physical before attempting to exercise. Jumping into training without knowing why you are in pain and perhaps making it worse can lead to serious injuries. You need to be strong (Jackson, 2016b) if you are unable to do the most basic of the calisthenics exercises you will not be able to progress onto the more difficult exercises. Talk to a personal trainer or physiotherapist to help you build up the strength needed to start this kind of training. The same can be said for mobility, if you cannot move your body through the movements required then you will struggle through them. Take the time to increase your shoulder mobility with stretching or basic exercises before moving on. No one needs a torn rotator cuff in their shoulder. The shoulder isn't the only place that takes a lot of strain. Calisthenics is tough on your joints so for the elderly this could be difficult, however, not impossible. Taking care of your joints is vital to your health in the future so do take the time to recover between training days and eating a good diet.

Now for the elephant in the room: Physical impairment. There are many different kinds of impairments that can be seen in people, and this does limit the number of exercises that can be done with calisthenics without injury. However, do not let this stop you for a moment! You might not be able to do all the possible movement patterns, especially for someone who is a paraplegic, who would still have amazing upper body strength, but many beginner exercises can work on other parts of your body. Even if you are recovering from a serious injury there are some exercises that are aimed at helping you regain a form that you can use to get stronger (Disability Horizons, 2016).

Lastly, we have old injuries. They pain us when it rains or just pain us in general. Old injuries are weaknesses but they are not something that can sentence us to stay away from any form of exercise unless stated so by a doctor. You need to strengthen the affected area until it is able to get a decent workout once more. This is something that takes time and it shouldn't be taken alone. Speaking with doctors to find the right medicine, diet, or training regime is a sure way to take an old injury and turn it into a weakness that you can work on to improve your body. It just needs time and a good mindset, nothing is impossible if you set your mind to it.

At the end of the day injuries and becoming injured are something that is part and parcel of exercise. It cannot always be avoided but we can do our best to prevent something serious by taking the time to know how to do the exercises correctly, warming up and cooling down, taking the time to do the research, and lastly, knowing what we can and can't do. It is also important to realize that when injured you need to take the time to heal, progression can wait, the quicker you heal correctly the faster you can get back to form. Taking a rest and recovering is as important as training, you just need the right mindset to realize that. Don't give up, do the physiotherapy, get back your base strength then move forward. And even if you can't move forward, take a step back, re-evaluating where you are in your training, and try again. The training will always be there tomorrow, no need to rush.

8

MEGA MOVEMENT PATTERNS

L et's have a quick recap: Calisthenics is the use of one's own weight to get a workout which is achieved through using the body's own natural movement patterns (Live Well Team, 2019), actions we perform without thinking about it, i.e. bending over or squatting to pick up something that has fallen. Some people refer to this as functional movement patterns. All movements follow a certain pattern. When you raise your arm it isn't just one muscle doing the work, it is several and they activate in a certain sequence (Woodruff, 2003) depending on how you raise your arm, be it in front of you or towards the side. These movements can be either normal or abnormal, which could be due to injury or taught behavior such as limping even after the injury has healed. Self-taught abnormal movements are often caused when the brain is trying to protect us from pain, reminding us that a certain movement hurts, even well after the injury has recovered. The brain needs to be retrained with the correct movement pattern to stop abnormal movement patterns from developing and staying with us in the future as that can cause more harm than good. This is why a good attitude to training is vital when it comes to practicing the movement patterns. Thinking 'I can't' because of an old injury is going to cause you to try to use other muscles to compensate and that is not what you want. In calisthenics the movement patterns are precise and activate certain muscle groups to complete them, activating the wrong muscles means your form is not correct and you will not be able to do the training correctly. Your mindset plays a vital role, let's change the 'I can't' to I'm going to take it nice and slow'.

Why are movement patterns important to people? We are designed to move (McCall, n.d.), not sit still for endless hours every day. Movement causes multiple sets of muscles to work together, influencing what the next set does during something as simple as walking or as intense as training. Being active allows your joints a wider range of motion. A mobile joint means fewer injuries while training. Non-movement can cause muscles to atrophy and make movement so difficult it can result in injury or needing intervention by medically trained professionals. It is for this reason that mobility can be enhanced with the use of exercises that work closely with movement patterns.

Of the various kinds of movements, our bodies can do, there are five basic movement patterns that we can follow: Pushing, pulling, single-sides, rotational, and bending (Greenblatt, 2016). Each of these movements is important as they are the base of calisthenics. Twisting exercises aim to work on the lower back and stomach muscles together and prevent you from solely letting those back muscles do all the heavy lifting. This movement is seen when you are throwing a ball. The twisting can be trained in two ways, either as allowing the rotation to happen, as seen with a V-sit twist, or resisting the rotation (anti-rotation), as seen with the one arm plank (Perry, 2020). Pushing and pulling are self-explanatory. It is the ability to bring something closer to you and the ability to move something away from you. Something as simple as opening and closing a door is an example of using the push and pull movement pattern. Bending over is likely one of our most important movement sets as it allows us to pick up anything that has fallen below our hip height. However, people get lazy when it comes to picking things up and they tend to bend at the waist, then wonder why their backs are always hurting. A slight bend at the hips and using the legs to go down (a squat if you will) and back up is the correct way to do this movement set. Then we have single-sided movements, usually for stepping over something, which requires a person to have not only balance but also flexibility in their movements. It is likely when you are using these exercises that you will notice if one side of your body is weaker than the other and will be able to work on it. Walking Lunges are a great way to train this movement pattern as it forces you to think about your balance as well as powering your legs. Perry (2020) also makes mention of the gait movement pattern, which is a combination of pulling, twisting, and lunging, simply put, it is your ability to walk forward, at whatever pace you want.

Those are your five, or six if you include gait, basic movement patterns that our bodies generally follow every single day. We already know these, we don't need someone to teach it to us but we need them to be able to do any exercises.

THE MAIN CALISTHENIC MOVEMENT PATTERNS

Once you have a basic understanding of our natural movement patterns you will start to understand how calisthenics is actually good for us and builds on what we already have available to us. You don't need to be able to Bench Press 100 lbs to start, you just need to know how to do a basic Push-Up, and not even on your toes, one on knees is good enough to start with. With knowing the basic movement patterns you are now able to use them to understand the major movement patterns used for calisthenics. The information for this section is taken from Maximum Potential Calisthenics (n.d.), Walker (2016), Kavadlo (2018), and Robles & Robles (2020).

Push

The push movement is divided into two categories: horizontal (flat) and vertical (upright). The horizontal push aims to move weight away from the front of you. The most common exercises here are the various types of Push-Ups and horizontal presses that work on the chest and tricep muscles. The vertical push is about pushing the weight away from you but not towards your front but rather over your head. The muscles that are targeted with these kinds of movements are your shoulders, traps, and triceps as well as your core, depending on the exercises that you choose to do. Exercises like Handstand Push-Ups and vertical presses aim to use this movement pattern.

Pull

Similar to the push movement, the pull movement can also be divided into vertical and horizontal movements. The horizontal movements aim to pull the weight towards you. Any form of rowing, seated or standing, is a great exercise to help with this movement. If you have a rowing machine or like to use one this likely is the easiest of the gym equipment to use if you do not like weights. The muscles that get the workout from this are the rhomboids and the spinal erectors. The vertical pull is where you are pulling a weight vertically in relation to your body. With this type of movement, your lats and biceps are doing all the work. Exercises that are great for the vertical pull include the Plank Rows and Pull-Ups.

Because the push and pull movements are so different and exercise unique muscle groups it is a good idea to find a balance between the two of them to allow for maximum development across the arms, back and chest. The exercises listed here are by no means the only ones available but are the most commonly known ones. When designing your exercise regime do the research to see which are the best exercises for your capability.

Squat

Squats are a type of movement known as knee flexion exercises, where you are only moving along a vertical axis (up and down). This is an important exercise for the lower back and legs as it exercises the posterior and anterior muscles in them. Many muscles have to work together to get the perfect Squat and these are quadriceps, hamstrings, glutes, in the legs as well as hip flexors (a set of muscles that allow the hip to flex), spinal erectors, abdominals (in the core). This is a great pattern to learn as it helps with stiffness in the spine as well as stability. The common Squat is the go-to for this movement pattern but there are many other varieties that you can try such as the Split-Squat and the Walking Lunge.

Forward Flexion (Anterior Chain)

The forward flexion is the bending of the body towards your feet, concentrating on the abdominal muscles, and though the variety of sit-ups is something that uses this movement pattern some of the exercises, such as Hanging Leg Raises does need equipment that allows you to hang and thus makes use of other muscles such as lats, biceps, triceps, and deltoids.

Hinge (Posterior Chain)

The hinge is the counterpart to the forward flexion and works on the posterior set of muscles rather than the anterior. Weakened posterior muscles will have an influence on your posture so be sure to work out your front and back. Many forms of Bridging, Deadlifts, and Kettlebell Swings aim to work your entire posterior chain of muscles, from the back of your shoulders down into the back of your legs.

The anterior and the posterior chains must be trained together as not to cause any imbalances. The reason for this is that over time an imbalance of these muscles can cause a shift in the bones as one set of muscles can pull too strongly in one direction (Furness, 2017) and can lead to chronic pain problems. Be mindful of this as you set up your own training regime.

Lateral Chain

The lateral chain of muscles can be found at the sides of your body, muscles such as your obliques (abdomen), lats, lateral deltoids, spinal erectors (back), and the muscles on the side of your legs. Some of these muscles are found in already mentioned muscle groups (or chains) but to purely exercise just those lateral muscles you need to employ the Side Plank or the Human Flag (Red Delta Project, n.d.) isometrically, first right then left, or vice versa, your choice. The importance of training your lateral chain is that it plays a vital role in having your upper body and lower muscles work together.

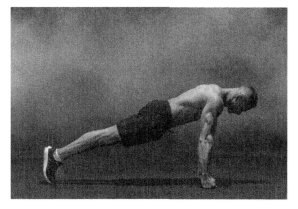

*Man preparing for a Push-Up showing well-developed
lateral chain muscles.*

DESIGNING YOUR OWN MOVEMENT PATTERNS ROUTINE

Now that you are almost at the end of the book, you have
learned a lot about calisthenics, from the importance of diet and
sleep all the way to the type of movements that are required by
the various types of exercises. With this knowledge, you are
now able to come up with your own routine for your training
session. If you are not comfortable with designing your own
training session yet, don't worry! Kuslikis (n.d.-b) has a
wonderful website called *A Shot of Adrenaline* which offers
free (yes, free) training programs for beginners of calisthenics.
These programs even include step by step pictures as well as
warm-ups and cool-downs for each day that you work out on.
However, before starting any exercise regime there are some
things that need to be considered.

The first is your personal objectives. What do you want from exercise? If you are not sure of what you want then you cannot begin anything. Remember the journal back in chapter 4? This is going to be your starting point. Your goal is where you start. Once that is in place you can build up around it.

After you have your objectives you need to work on the variation of the patterns you will be using for your training. Robles & Robles (2020) use seven different movement patterns in their training guide. The first is for the chest and triceps, then working with the pulling movement pattern concentrating on the back, then the vertical pushing for the shoulders, squats for concentrating on the legs, then single-side training for coordination and balance, then glute-hip extensions (bridges), and finally, abs. From there they tell the reader to design a training program as follows: Choose one exercise from each chapter (seven in total). Of those seven, choose between 2-3 to do per training session. You can decide how you want the training to be—either a full-body workout or a split body workout. Each exercise should have between 8-15 repetitions per set which can be between 2-4. If you are unable to complete 8 reps for all the sets then the exercise is too difficult and you have to regress the exercise to an earlier form. For example, Push-Ups on your toes regress to incline Push-Ups or even Push-Ups on the knees. If you can complete 12-15 reps easily then you need to progress the exercise to a higher level. Following this, you can train whenever you want but they suggest not training longer than 20 minutes at a time.

There are advantages and disadvantages to using a premade exercise plan or making one yourself. The plans by Kuslikis (n.d.-b) vary from 5-6 exercises per training session, of which there are five sessions over five days and they cover the entire body if you do all five days. With a concentration on individual muscle groups, chest and triceps, lower body, back, core, shoulders, and biceps, missing a single day of training can result in a certain muscle group lagging behind. Though this can be a disadvantage it is by no means a negative if you as the person training can stick to the training session with perseverance. A great advantage for this author is that his site has links to videos to show you how to do the correct form for most of the exercises. A full-body training session also has its disadvantages of which one is the recovery period, about 48 hours (Better Health, n.d.), required to allow you to rest effectively between training sessions.

Designing your own training program can be very difficult, especially if you are not honest with yourself about your capabilities. Everyone would love to be able to show off that perfect Handstand Push-Up but how many of us can even do a Handstand unassisted? It is advised to rather look at the most basic of the exercises and try them for a few sessions before moving the bar higher. It is always better to start at the bottom and work yourself up to the higher levels. Remember, calisthenic practices, especially the higher leveled exercises, require two things. The first is that you know the basics and the second is that you have worked on your base strength while trying to achieve the perfect form. If you cannot control the muscle groups associated with a particular movement pattern, you will hurt yourself.

This is why research is crucial. Kuslikis (n.d.-b) is by no means the only person who shares exercises on the internet. Resources like YouTube are great for finding out what the exercise is, as some names are strange and don't accurately describe the exercise, and show you the correct form. Take the time to research everything and make sure you can complete the exercises with the correct form. If you cannot, regress it. Robles & Robles (2020) show the progression of all their exercises and have photos to show you the correct form. If you are still unable to complete the easiest of the move sets perhaps speak to a personal trainer that could help you. Or, if you don't want to spend too much money, ask a friend to spot you while you try the exercises so that they can help you achieve the correct form.

As you are planning the program don't be too overzealous. Don't put too much on yourself for your first, second, or third training sessions. Take it slow but consider the duration of time you want to spend doing exercise. You are, after all, still a busy person that needs to do things outside of training. The NHS (2019c) states that an adult between the ages of 19 and 64 should be getting strength exercises up to two times a week, along with 150 minutes of moderate exercise, heart rate of 70 percent of your maximum, or 75 minutes of vigorous exercise, 70-85 percent of maximum (Mayo Clinic, 2019a). Keep this in mind as you are designing your own regime. And don't forget your warm-up and cool down! A total of 5-10 minutes is suffi-cient for getting the muscles warm and then cooling them down afterward. Try aiming for a 30-minute training session with enough time to do a decent warm-up and cool down, plus don't forget to do those stretches. If this is too much then try Robles & Robles' (2020) approach of only a 20-minute session and slowly build it up until you can do a longer workout. Workouts can be increased and decreased by looking at how many reps are done in each set as well as how many sets are being done. When designing your training program don't forget to include recovery times during the sets as well as during the session. You may feel great after two or three days of training but you do not want the fun to grow boring and to feel tired and sore all the time.

The last thing to consider is how many sessions you will have in a week. This depends on whether you want to do a full-body workout or a split workout. As you will need more recovery from a full-body workout you will maybe get 2-3 training days at most, whereas the split training will allow for more days training but you will only get your own body trained across 2-3 sessions instead of one. That is something that you will need to consider.

Sara Lindberg (2020) suggests that for cardio you train about five days in total if you are doing 30 minutes of moderate cardio training, or three times a week at 25 minutes of vigorous cardio training, or even two days of each to aid in weight loss. She also suggests about 2-3 days of full-body strength training for a beginner. As you improve you can try 3-4 days of the split type sessions where you can divide it into the upper and lower body or any other split you would prefer, i.e. push and pull. Those that are more advanced in their training can train 4-5 days with a similar split as seen with the intermediate level, though their week could be structured to allow a single day's rest in the middle of the training days to allow for a total of two days rest throughout the whole week. This is only one suggestion of many you could find; at the end of the day you need to find what is right for your body and you. Remember, if you stick to a training program you will reach your goals in the end. Don't forget to reward yourself for reaching your various goals and have fun. Once you are no longer having fun, there is no point.

9

OVER 30 CALISTHENIC WORKOUTS TO DO AT HOME

D o not start the book here! Please take the time to go to the front of the book to learn more about calisthenics before trying any of the exercises listed below. Consider making a goal and keeping a diary to help with achieving what you are setting out to do. The exercises listed below are just some of the examples to train the various muscle groups of your body. If they do not suit your needs do not hesitate in scouring the internet, or the references at the end of this book, to find more and exciting challenges. The below exercises were gathered from many sources such as (Kuslikis, n.d.-b), Bhanot (2017), Eisinger (2017), Mercedes (2019), Robles & Robles (2020), and Tucker *et al.* (2020).

Once more, please consult your doctor before starting any new kind of training program or diet and be wary of your own capabilities. Now that that is out of the way let's get started with some calisthenics.

WARM-UPS AND COOL-DOWNS

No training program is complete without warm-ups and cool-downs, so do aim to add them to your training program to aid in less sore muscles the next day. Swinging your arms in small or large circles, or forward and back across the chest, helps for stretching and warming up the chest and triceps. Stretches for these muscles include the Door Frame stretch over the Overhead Elbow stretch. Stretches are only held for a few seconds while movements are done for about 10 reps. For your legs, you can use Knee Hugs, standing or sitting Quad stretches, or the Butterfly stretch. If you are particularly flexible try for some Toe Touches, but don't force it—it needs to be a slow stretch down and back up. For your back try some yoga stretches like the Cat Stretch pose or Trunk Twisting to loosen all the muscles up. To help the core muscles try some Side Bends or the Cobra Stretch pose. For those shoulders and biceps try the Forearm Stretch, Arm Crosses, and some Shoulder stretches, using a wall to help you get the right stretch. You can also make use of a brisk walk, or doing one or two sets of your planned exercises for the day done slowly, to get a nice warm-up in. Don't feel limited by what is stated here.

CHEST WORKOUTS

Beginner

Push-Ups are difficult, especially if your form isn't good, but don't fret. This is an excellent all-body training exercise so you can start with something like the Wall Push-Up, which helps you keep the right form, to move onto the more advanced Push-Ups later. Remember that a Push-Up at this level will have your hands at shoulder width for the best form.

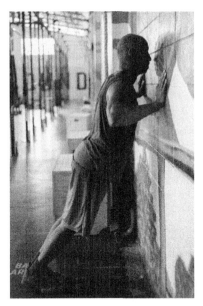

Man doing a Wall Push-Up.

From a Wall Push-Up, you can progress to an incline Push-Up. This is where you are doing a Push-Up on a flat surface that is raised. Start at chair height, or counter if you feel you aren't ready, and steadily move downwards in height until you are completing a full Push-Up on the ground. Remember to keep your body as straight as possible and don't dip the hips or arch the back. Keep a good tempo when going down and coming back up and breathe!

Intermediate

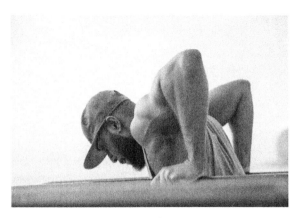

Man doing Chest Dips.

From here the variety of Push-Ups are many. While flat on the ground, you can bring your hands together for the Close-grip Push-Up, which is less than shoulder-width or even with hands touching. Or you can spread your hands apart for the Wide Push-Ups, which is further than your shoulder width, and that will change which muscles you are concentrating on. From here you can move onto the Decline Push-Up where your feet are raised on a bench, this is great for a chest workout. Chest Dips, unlike conventional Dips, need your shoulders to be quite stable as you will be using your entire body weight to move up and down.

BACK WORKOUTS

Beginner

You will get no other exercise quite as good for your back as a Pull-Up, but they are tough to do, so before you start looking for a door frame to do a Pull-Up, try breaking it down into easier exercises first. A Wall Pull is your starting point. Find a doorway that you can train in, and make sure the side you are holding cannot be slipped from easily and cause you injury. Bring your feet close to the wall you are holding and lean back until your arms are fully extended. Once you are fully extended, concentrate on pulling yourself back up to a standing position using only your arms, then return to the extended position—that was one rep. This can be modified by using a box or raised surface with the Pull-Up bar. Stand on the box and grip the bar, lower your feet from the box, and slowly descend—this is called a Negative Pull-Up. From here you can even keep your feet slightly in front of you and use the Feet Assisted Pull-Up. From here the Chin-Up is next. The difference between a Pull-Up and a Chin-Up is how you grip the bar. Palms gripping outwards for a Pull-Up and gripping inward for a Chin-Up.

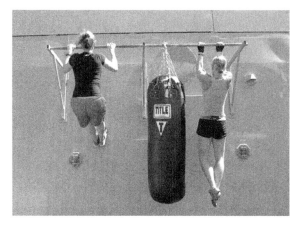

Pull-Up on left and Chin-Up on right.

If Pull-Ups seem a distant dream of yours don't feel limited by them. Try some Superman or Aquaman exercises to help develop those back muscles. Both exercises start the same: lie on your stomach with your arms extended. With Supermans, raise your legs and arms simultaneously with your head remaining down, and hold the position for a few seconds, then return to rest. With the Aquaman exercise, you raise one leg with the opposing arm as high as possible before bringing the next set up, and this will almost give you the appearance of paddling.

Intermediate

Once you have the basic Pull-Up under control, you can try moving your hands to a closer, Close-Hands Pull-Ups, or wider position, Wide Pull-Ups, to get more from your back muscles working. If you want to add some core strengthening to your Pull-Ups you can make use of the L-Pull-Up where your legs are bent at a 90 degrees position in relation to your arms. The closer your hands are to one another, the more of a workout your arms get; the further apart they are, the more of a workout your back will get, especially your lats.

SHOULDER WORKOUTS

Beginner

There is no better way to develop your shoulders than the Pike Push-Up, and like the previous Push-Up variations, there are several steps to this before you can complete the full Pike Push-Up. A Pike position needs to have a V-shape where the head is down, so start on the knees, keeping the back level before lowering your head to the ground and pushing upwards. This is a kneeling Pike Push-Up. The next level is the Incline Pike Push-Up. Place your hands on a chair to help you get the same action as what you practiced in the knee position. Similar to the Incline Push-Up, you can lower the height until you are performing the Pike Push-Ups with your hands on the floor and achieving the V-shape by raising onto the tips of your toes with the buttocks in the air.

Intermediate

As if Pike Push-Ups weren't difficult enough, let's make them more so. By bringing your hands closer together, instead of at shoulder width, you can get more of a shoulder workout. You can increase the amount of weight you have on your shoulders by using the Decline Pike Push-Up. You can do this by raising your feet onto a chair or bench, maintaining the V-shape. Please be careful when doing this as you do not want the chair to slide out from under you. Make sure that all surfaces you use are stable. The last of the intermediate exercises is in preparation for the coveted Handstand Push-Up. You will need assistance here or at least a sturdy wall. To do a Handstand Hold, get into a Handstand position against a wall and hold it. Try to hold the position for longer and longer periods to build up your shoulder strength. Make sure your core muscles are tight to maintain this form correctly.

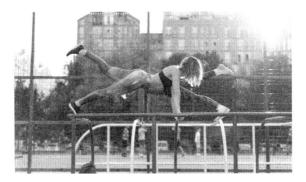

A pair of trainees making use of a metal frame to work on their arms, shoulders, legs, back, and abdominal muscles.

AB WORKOUTS

Beginner

When you hear the phrase "ab workout," most people immediately think of Sit-Ups and Crunches; though they can help, these are not your only option. Like the Push-Up that activates many sets of muscles, the Plank is sure to get you sweating and possibly swearing to complete. There is nothing simpler to a Plank, sorry to say, though there are quite a few varieties to this exercise. A typical Plank position is done on the forearms, though some people like to stand in a Push-Up position to get the same effect, with the shoulder causing a 90-degree bend with the forearm, and on your toes.

If you want something a little easier to get those abdominal muscles engaged try the Lying Bent Knee Raise. You lie flat on your back, raise your legs a little off the ground to activate the abdominal muscles, then bring your knees towards your chest and hold it there for a second or two before relaxing to the starting position again. If this is too easy, instead of bringing your knees to your chest, keep your legs straight and raise them perpendicular to your body, which can be done with both legs or one at a time. This is called a Leg Raise, and doing this slowly will allow for maximum abdominal engagement. A variety of this exercise can also be done in the gym with the use of a Roman Chair where you are vertical instead of horizontal. You can bring either your knees to your chest or raise your extended legs to be perpendicular to your hanging body; these are called Hanging Knee or Leg Raises.

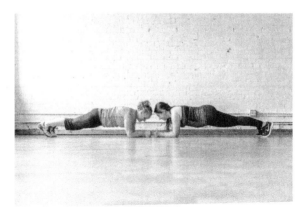

Activating the core by planking.

A great combination of ab exercises is combining Bicycle Kicks, Flutters, Leg Holds, and Windscreen Wipers. For the Bicycle Kicks lie on your back and move your legs as if you are pushing the pedals of a bicycle. Flutters are the same as kicking in the pool if you are swimming Freestyle, except you are on your back for this exercise. Leg Holds are the start of your Leg Raises, except your heels remain only a few inches above the ground and don't go further. With Windscreen Wipers you raise your legs a little above the ground and have them cross over each other back and forth, just like the windscreen wipers of your car. Ten reps each, 10-second leg hold, with about three sets is enough to make you well aware of your stomach muscles. If you really want a challenge don't set your heels on the ground at any stage during the set.

Intermediate

Can ab workouts get more difficult? Yes, yes they can. A Side Plank is a great way to target your lateral chain of muscles. From a regular Plank position, you use one of your arms to reach for the heavens and hold that position for a few seconds before returning to your starting position. Don't forget to do both sides. Any variety of Plank that requires you to raise an arm or arm-leg combination is something that will also make your stomach muscles scream for a break, so don't forget to breathe. If you want to add extra weight to the Plank to strengthen your arms, you can do this by making use of a chair to make a Decline Plank or add weight items to your mid-back for the regular Plank.

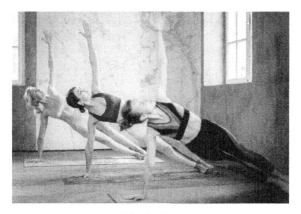

Side planking.

ARM WORKOUTS

Intermediate

Your arm muscles have been targeted by quite a few previously mentioned exercises, so these exercises will be upgrades to the basics that have already been done. Plank Taps are great for arms and abdominals. Get into a Push-Up position and raise one hand to tap the opposite shoulder, and repeat with the other hand—that is a single repetition. Since you are already in the Push-Up position, why not try the Plank Up-Down? With one arm at a time go down into a Plank position and then return to a Push-Up position—that is one rep. Bench Dips can be done by setting your hands against the edge of a bench and dipping downwards by bending your elbows and coming back up. Do not lock your elbows. For extra resistance try holding the Dip for a few seconds before coming back up. A Diamond Push-Up is what you are left with when your Close-Hand Push-Up eventually meets in the middle, and it gives you a great deltoid workout. If you have a very sturdy, high table, you can even try Inverted Rows with your knees bent. Get under the table and grip the edge, keeping your feet on the ground and your body horizontal to it, pull yourself up, keeping your elbows tucked in, then lower yourself once more.

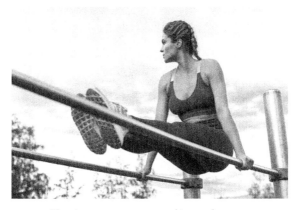

Here is a young woman working on her core.

LEG WORKOUTS

Beginner

You are spoiled for choice when it comes to leg exercises. Squats are the go-to exercise for the beginner, but be sure not to arch your back, and keep your heels firmly on the ground to get the most benefit from this training. A level up from a standard Squat is the Jumping Squat. Concentrate on how you land so as not to injure your ankles. Start in a Squat position then jump upwards with as much power as you can from your legs then land in a Squat position again. Lunges are a great way to get a little cardio in, as you can do them by walking forward or by doing the Lunges forward, backward, or diagonally to work all the leg muscles. Concentrate on stepping forward, or in a preferred direction, and lowering your knee to almost touching the floor, then stepping back, which is powered by the leg that stepped forward. Follow the action with the other leg. Concentrate on your abs while doing this as controlled abs help with the balance that could be lost. If you want to add a step of difficulty here you can combine the forward, backward, and diagonal Lunges and not return your forward stepping leg to the center but step back into a Backward Lunge immediately. If you do this consider completing all the reps on one leg before moving on to the reps of the second leg to complete the set. With Calf Raises you just need something to steady yourself as you raise yourself to your toes and back down. Varieties of this include the Single Calf Raise, working on a raised surface, or lowering yourself below your starting point, which can be achieved when you are standing on a stair. Try not to do these exercises too fast as you want all the muscles to engage.

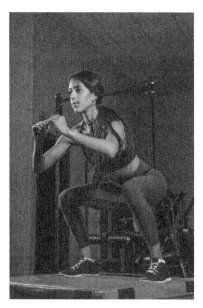

Squatting with perfect form.

Intermediate

Once your leg muscles are stronger you can try Wall Sits, which is a Squat with your back against a wall and you hold it for as long as possible. It will burn but do not continue if there is pain. Then there are the Box Jumps, but be warned, there needs to be an element of coordination and athleticism here as you will be required to jump onto a stable surface. Do not make this too high as you can hurt yourself attempting to do this.

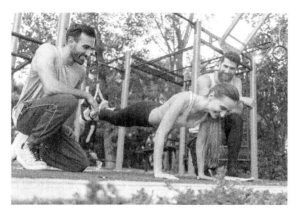

*Some exercises can be tough so remember to make use
of workout partners to help you out.*

BECOMING AN EXPERT

Becoming an expert in calisthenics is no easy matter as it requires dedication to the beginner and intermediate levels before you can even start anything as difficult as a handstand Push-Up, Dragon Flags, or even Planches. One-handed and Clapping Push-Ups are great exercises that work on arms, core, and back. Planche is the advanced version of planking where your feet no longer touch the ground. The Typewriter Pull-Up requires you to not only pull your weight up but also to move from left to right, or vice versa, once at the top before returning to the center and going back down to attempt it again. Then there are the Pistol Squats where you are required to go all the way down to the ground on one leg, while the other is held out in front of you, before attempting to get back to a standing position. All these exercises sound amazing yet absolutely daunting —and they should, as this is what you will achieve if you continue with your training.

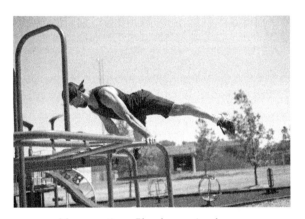

Man executing a Planche on a jungle gym.

Cover your basics, work on your strength, go through beginner and intermediate levels before even attempting the start of the advanced exercises, and remember if you cannot do it then regress to something easier and try again. Training is what makes you stronger, not jumping to the most difficult of the exercises.

KEEPING A TRAINING DIARY

Since you have a goal diary why not extend on it by keeping your training in there as well? You can write down your training programs and even keep pictures in the book of what you are doing to remind you what the correct form looks like. It becomes easier to visualize yourself growing if you are able to look back on what you have done. Don't be afraid to mix and match different types of training either. If you want to do some cardio like jogging or cycling work it into your training program but do not overwork yourself or get bored. Set your diary up in such a way that you can plan for a week in advance so that you can mentally prepare yourself for the challenges you are going to face. You do not have to do any of this alone. Consider getting a partner to work out with you who will both be an encouragement and allow for some friendly competition. Make the diary into a contract; once your week has been planned you have to stick to what you have written down. Don't be scared to reward yourself after your hard work. You deserve a break after working so hard. Once a week of training is completed, plan your next week, or even your next month. Keep moving forward!

CONCLUSION

We all want to be healthy and fit, and for some, it seems like a daunting task but it isn't. You don't need expensive gym memberships or bulky gym equipment, you just need yourself. That bodyweight you are trying to lose is going to help you do it. Calisthenics aims to use that weight to give you the workout of your life. Exercise goes hand in hand with sleep and a good diet so don't forget to take a careful look at what you place on your plate in the future. Basically, if it comes in a box or can, be wary of it. However, don't throw away all your "junk food," take the time to consider your diet and see where you can improve to allow for the best possible you. Sleeping poorly will cause problems in both your diet and exercise, so make sure you are getting good quality sleep every night. Staring at that poster of the perfect body isn't going to get you anywhere, so set up a big goal with several smaller goals to allow you to feel the journey towards your main goal, but be wary of your own capabilities. To get the most from calisthenics keep a diary of all your exercises, targets, or full-body workouts, and don't forget to take those before and after picture so that you can see how you've progressed, not just in inches but also in the varying difficulty levels. Calisthenics is both a progressive and regressive type of exercise. You are building up towards those expert levels but if you do not build your strength and form for the beginner level, you will be doing more regressive forms than progressive forms. Lastly, have fun, play around with the exercises presented in the book, or look for your own online. You are in charge of creating and sticking to your own training regime. All of this is up to you as you have now been armed with the knowledge of calisthenics. Get those diaries out and start your research.

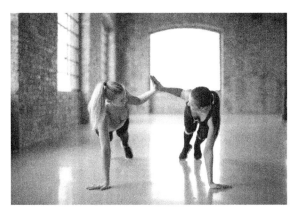

Training buddies makes exercise so much fun.

A SPECIAL GIFT TO OUR READERS

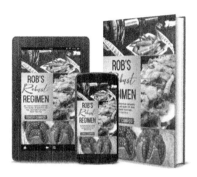

Included with your purchase of this book is a copy of Rob's Robust Regimen, to help you get started on your health and fitness journey and inspire you to create your own similar regimen to get where you want to be.

Click the link below and let us know which email address to deliver it to.

www.yourfinefettle.com

REFERENCES

272447. (2015, April, 17). *Pull-Up on left and chin-up on right*. Pixabay.

https://pixabay.com/photos/fitness-workout-exercise-females-725881/

8fit Team. (n.d.). *Training differences: Men and women.*

https://8fit.com/fitness/training-differences-men-and-women/

Aimee. (n.d.). *"Good food" and "bad food".* Center for Discovery.

https://centerfordiscovery.com/blog/good-food-bad-food/

Andy. (2018, August, 28). *Why is it good to go to a gym?* Broffice.

https://broffice.org/why-is-it-good-to-go-to-a-gym/

Aragona, M., Barbato, A., Cavani, A., Costanzo, G., & Mirisola, C. (2020). Negative impacts of COVID-19 lockdown on mental health service access and follow-up adherence for immigrants and individuals in socio-economic difficulties. *Public Health*, 186, 52–56. https://doi.org/10.1016/j.puhe.2020.06.055

Araújo, P. (2019, October, 25). *Man performing a Handstand Push-Up*. Unsplash.

https://unsplash.com/photos/VMsjpnB21hQ

Associated Press. (2020, March, 21). *Man runs marathon on 7-metre balcony during French lockdown*. The Guardian.

https://www.theguardian.com/world/2020/mar/21/man-runs-marathon-on-7-metre-balcony-during-french-lockdown

Bender, N. (2017, February 10). *You asked: Which is more important: Sleep, diet or exercise?* Vital Record.

https://vitalrecord.tamhsc.edu/you-asked-which-is-more-important-sleep-diet-or-exercise/

Better Health. (n.d.). *Resistance training: Health benefits.* Better Health.

https://www.betterhealth.vic.gov.au/health/healthyliving/resistance-training-health-benefits

Bhanot, S. (2017, October, 11). *10 exercises for a stronger back you can do at home without any equipment.* Scoop Whoop.

https://www.scoopwhoop.com/back-exercises-without-equipment/

Bode, L. (2003). *Avoid common fitness pitfalls.* Top End Sports.

https://www.topendsports.com/fitness/program-pitfalls.htm

Borodinova, V. (2014, June, 14). *The sad setback of an injury.* Pexels.

https://www.pexels.com/photo/young-sad-woman-with-broken-leg-on-sofa-4497828/

Bowerman, S. (n.d.). Calories: *Why drastic cutting may backfire.* Discover Good Nutrition, Fitness & Beauty.

https://discovergoodnutrition.com/2016/09/cutting-calories/

Brazier, Y. (2018, February, 12). *Calories: Recommended intake, burning calories, tips, and daily needs.* Medical News Today.

https://www.medicalnewstoday.com/articles/245588

CDC. (2020a, September, 8). *Heart disease facts & statistics.*

https://www.cdc.gov/heartdisease/facts.htm

CDC. (2020b, September, 17). *The health effects of overweight and obesity.*

https://www.cdc.gov/healthyweight/effects/index.html

Ceban, A. (2019, June, 2). *Man preparing to do a Pistol Squat.* Pixabay.

https://pixabay.com/photos/fitness-healthy-gym-exercise-4245628/

Chicago Tribune. (2018, January, 16). *Four crucial ways that sleep helps the body to heal.* https://www.chicagotribune.com/ suburbs/advertising/marketplace/ct-ss-suburbs-four-crucial-ways-that-sleep-helps-the-body-to-heal-20180112dto-story.html

Coleman, E. (n.d.). *15 home workout mistakes to avoid.* Fit Father Project.

https://www.fitfatherproject.com/home-workout-mistakes/

Commonwealth Sports Club. (2015, August, 26). *Fresh vs. processed foods.*https://commonwealthsportsclub.com/fresh-vs-processed-foods/

Conner, S. (2017, January, 1). *7 best tips to use massage therapy as a source of injury prevention.* The Health Sessions.

https://thehealthsessions.com/massage-therapy-injury-prevention/

Cordier, A. (2018, February, 9). *5 reasons why warm up exercises are important.* Fit Athletic. https://fitathletic.com/5-reasons-warm-exercises-important/

Crockett, Z. (2019, January, 5). *Why gym memberships are a terrible investment.* The Hustle. https://thehustle.co/gym-membership-cost

Cronkleton, E. (2019a, September, 5). *Strength training at home: Workouts with and without equipment.* Heath Line.

https://www.healthline.com/health/exercise-fitness/strength-training-at-home

Cronkleton, E. (2019b, December, 17). *Cooldown exercises: 16 ways to cool down with instructions.* Healthline.

https://www.healthline.com/health/exercise-fitness/cooldown-exercises#for-seniors

Cronkleton, E. (2020, May, 29). *6 ways that being flexible benefits your health.* Healthline. https://www.healthline.com/health/benefits-of-flexibility

Cyborggainz. (2020, October, 6). *Calisthenics workout: How to avoid injuries.*https://cyborggainz.com/press/f/calisthenics-workout-how-to-avoid-injuries

De Khors, N. (n.d.). *Squatting with perfect form.* Burst.

https://burst.shopify.com/photos/squatting-exercise?q=squating

Delavier, F., & Gundill, M. (2012). *The strength training anatomy workout.* Human Kinetics.

Dellitt, J. (2018, March, 21). *6 ways to cope and stay positive with an injury.* Aaptiv.

https://aaptiv.com/magazine/stay-positive-with-an-injury

Disability Horizons. (2016, October, 20). *Disability sport: top 10 exercises for disabled people.* https://disabilityhorizons. com/2016/10/top-10-exercises-disabled-people/

Distelrath, M. (2019, March, 20) *Well defined calves.* Pixabay.

https://pixabay.com/photos/jog-run-sport-endurance-calves-4066243/

Eisinger, A. (2017, May, 9). *The 24 killer bodyweight moves for your butt.* Greatist.

https://greatist.com/move/bodyweight-butt-exercises

Ellis, P. (2020, April, 7). *8 common home workout mistakes to avoid while in quarantine.* Men's Health.

https://www.mh.co.za/workouts/8-common-home-workout-mistakes/

Fairytale, E. (2020, Feb, 28). *Side planking.* Pexels.

https://www.pexels.com/photo/women-practicing-yoga-3822187/

Frey, M. (2020, February, 13). *The benefits of a cool down after exercise.* Very Well Fit.

https://www.verywellfit.com/what-is-a-cool-down-3495457

Friedrich, C. (2019a, March, 26). *Pros and cons of training one body part per day.* Cathe. https://cathe.com/pros-and-cons-of-training-one-body-part-per-day/

Friedrich, C. (2019b, April, 14). *The pros and cons of full-body training routines.* Cathe.

https://cathe.com/the-pros-and-cons-of-full-body-training-routines/

Furness, P. (2017, August, 20). *Anterior and posterior chains.* Max Remedial.

https://maxremedial.com/blog/2017/8/16/anterior-and-posterior-chains

GMB Fitness. (2018, Jan, 17). *Man executing a planche on a jungle gym.* Unsplash. https://unsplash.com/photos/NYCVycvTbek

Grabowska, K. (2020, May, 9). *Remember to write everything down.* Pexels.

https://www.pexels.com/photo/crop-woman-taking-notes-in-diary-while-sitting-in-park-4497762/

Greenblatt, A. B. (2016, November, 9). *5 functional exercises to help your body move more efficiently.* Inquirer.

https://www.inquirer.com/philly/blogs/sportsdoc/5-
functional-exercises-to-help-your-body-move-efficiently.html

Guerra, J. (2017, December, 5). *How to reward yourself after a workout, according to experts.* Elite Daily.

https://www.elitedaily.com/p/how-to-reward-yourself-after-a-
workout-according-to-experts-6787768

Guerra, J. (2019, January, 29). *7 benefits of working out at home to keep in mind if gym sessions just aren't your scene.* Elite Daily.

https://www.elitedaily.com/p/7-benefits-of-working-out-at-
home-to-keep-in-mind-if-gym-sessions-just-arent-your-scene-
15904569

Harvard Health Publishing. (2013, October). *10 tips to prevent injuries when you exercise.*

https://www.health.harvard.edu/pain/10-tips-to-prevent-
injuries-when-you-exercise

Harvard Health Publishing. (2019, August, 20). *The 4 most important types of exercise.*https://www.health.harvard.edu/
exercise-and-fitness/the-4-most-important-types-of-exercise

Heathline. (2020, April, 30). *15 foods that boost the immune system.*

https://www.healthline.com/health/food-nutrition/foods-that-
boost-the-immune-system

Henry, M. (n.d.-a). *Women stretching after warm-up.* Burst.

https://burst.shopify.com/photos/women-stretching-in-exercise-class?q=Stretching%2C+exercise

Henry, M. (n.d.-b). *Activating the core by planking.* Burst.

https://burst.shopify.com/photos/two-women-planking-together?q=planking

Higgins, C. (2019, November, 27). *Bodyweight hamstring exercises: Hard like iron, flexible as a rope.* Calisthenics-Gear.

https://www.calisthenics-gear.com/bodyweight-hamstring-exercises/

Higgins, C. (2020, January, 3). *Calisthenics history: How calisthenics once ruled the schools and lost the battle to sports.* Calisthenics-Gear.

https://www.calisthenics-gear.com/calisthenics-history/

Holland, R. (n.d.). *6 essential mindsets for getting back in shape.* Breaking Muscle.

https://breakingmuscle.com/fitness/6-essential-mindsets-for-getting-back-in-shape

Huizen, J. (2019, January, 25). *Which foods can help you sleep?* Medical News Today.

https://www.medicalnewstoday.com/articles/324295

International Diabetes Federation. (2020, March, 25). *Home-based exercise for people with diabetes.*

https://www.idf.org/aboutdiabetes/what-is-diabetes/covid-19-and-diabetes/home-based-exercise.html

Jackson, D. (2016a, July, 24). *How to write a calisthenics program: Part 1.* School Of Calisthenics.

https://schoolofcalisthenics.com/2016/07/24/calisthenics-program/

Jackson, D. (2016b, September, 4). *5 things we wish we knew when starting calisthenics.* School Of Calisthenics.

https://schoolofcalisthenics.com/2016/09/04/starting-calisthenics/

Jackson, D. (n.d.-a). *Top 10 tips for beginners: Start today.* School Of Calisthenics.

https://schoolofcalisthenics.com/2017/02/19/start-calisthenics/

Jackson, D. (n.d.-b). *Setting effective goals (the difference between a dream and a goal).* School Of Calisthenics.

https://schoolofcalisthenics.com/2020/01/03/setting-effective-goals/

James, H. E. (n.d.). *10 real reasons we go to the gym.* Life Hack.

https://www.lifehack.org/315524/10-real-reasons-the-gym

Jones, O. (2020a, September, 17). *Muscles of the pectoral region.* Teach Me Anatomy.

https://teachmeanatomy.info/upper-limb/muscles/pectoral-region/

Jones, O. (2020b, October, 29). *The superficial back muscles, attachments, actions.* Teach Me Anatomy. https://teachmeanatomy.info/back/muscles/superficial/

Jurča, P. (2017, June, 8). *Well defined posterior muscles with no bulking.* Pixabay.

https://pixabay.com/photos/fitness-muscles-back-strengthening-2378993/

Kaiser, S., Engeroff, T., Niederer, D., Wurm, H., Vogt, L., &Banzer, W. (2018). The epidemiological profile of calisthenics athletes. *Deutsche Zeitschrift Für Sportmedizin,* 2018, 299–304. https://doi.org/10.5960/dzsm.2018.342

Kavadlo, D. (2018, October, 24). *7 movements you need for full-body strength.* BodyBuilding. https://www.bodybuilding.com/content/7-movements-you-need-for-full-body-strength.html

Kelly, C. (2016, November, 25). *Benefits of exercising at home: fitness gallery exercise equipment.* Fitness Gallery.

https://www.fitnessgallery.com/blog/exercise-tips/benefits-of-exercising-at-home/

Khicher, D. (2017, November, 16) *Well defined anterior muscles with no bulking.* Pixabay. https://pixabay.com/photos/biceps-triceps-fit-fitness-muscle-2945912/

King, C. (2019, March, 29). *A super quick and easy guide to calisthenics diet and supplements.* VoyedgeRX

https://www.voyedgerx.com/vrx-blog/2019/4/5/a-super-quick-and-easy-guide-to-calisthenics-diet-and-supplements

Kittaneh, F. (2015, August, 13). *Why food, sleep and exercise are critical to success.* Entrepreneur. https://www.entrepreneur.com/article/249387

Kunzler, D. (2020, June, 19). *Man with extreme flexibility.* Pixabay.

https://pixabay.com/photos/gymnast-dehnung-turner-gymnastics-5313469/

Kuslikis, T. (n.d.-a). *10 things I wish I knew about calisthenics skill achievement.* A Shot Of Adrenaline. https://ashotofadrenaline.net/calisthenics-skills/

Kuslikis, T. (n.d.-b). *Calisthenics for beginners: A complete 8-week workout program. body weight and calisthenics exercises & workouts.* A Shot Of Adrenaline.

https://ashotofadrenaline.net/calisthenics-for-beginners/?inf_contact_key=

28053b0a8cedbae0778595ddcf6c2f90459d0255b16dfcaa9646d76
d6fbd43e1#sheet

Langley, J. (2020, April, 19). *Don't make these 5 home workout mistakes.* JLPT.

https://langleypt.com/dont-make-these-5-home-workout-mistakes/

Legge, A. (n.d.). *The best way to train all 6 major muscle groups.* Legion Athletics.

https://legionathletics.com/muscle-groups/

Lindberg, S. (2020, May, 28). *How often should you work out: Legs, arms, abs, chest, and more.* Healthline.

https://www.healthline.com/health/how-often-should-you-work-out

Ling, T. (2020, November, 6). *New to home workouts? Don't make these 4 common mistakes.* Men's Health.

https://www.menshealth.com/uk/building-muscle/a754531/the-4-most-common-home-workout-mistakes/

Live Well Team. (2019, March, 22). *The 6 fundamental movement patterns.* Live Well Centre. https://livewellcentre.com/2019/03/22/the-6-fundamental-movement-patterns/

Lyda, J. (n.d.). *The benefits of calisthenics: 8 reasons to do bodyweight workouts.* Athletic Muscle. https://athleticmuscle. net/benefits-of-calisthenics/

Marcin, A. (2020, February, 25). *13 benefits of aerobic exercise.* Healthline.

https://www.healthline.com/health/fitness-exercise/benefits-of-aerobic-exercise

Maximum Potential Calisthenics. (n.d.). *Calisthenics fundamentals.*

https://www.mpcalisthenics.com/portfolio-items/calisthenics-fundamentals

Mayo Clinic. (2019a, August, 6). *Exercise intensity: How to measure it.*

https://www.mayoclinic.org/healthy-lifestyle/fitness/in-depth/exercise-intensity/art-20046887

Mayo Clinic. (2019b, August, 10). *Sleep disorders: Symptoms and causes.*

https://www.mayoclinic.org/diseases-conditions/sleep-disorders/symptoms-causes/syc-20354018

Mazzo, L. (2019, June, 14). *What is calisthenics (and should you be doing it)?* Shape.

https://www.shape.com/fitness/trends/what-is-calisthenics-workout-benefits

McCall, P. (n.d.). *Understanding mobility and the importance of movement preparation.* 24 Life.

https://www.24life.com/understanding-mobility-and-the-importance-of-movement-preparation/

Mercedes. (2019, March, 18). *Bodyweight chest workout for women.* Spot Me Girl.

https://heyspotmegirl.com/workout/chest/bodyweight-chest-workout-for-women/

Muscle Fit Pro. (2019, October, 26). *6 great reasons to start exercising.* Muscle Fit Pro.

https://www.musclefitpro.com/fitness/6-great-reasons-to-start-exercising/

NHS. (2019a, October, 8). *Physical activity guidelines for children (under 5 years).* https://www.nhs.uk/live-well/exercise/physical-activity-guidelines-children-under-five-years/

NHS. (2019b, October, 8). *Physical activity guidelines for children and young people.* https://www.nhs.uk/live-well/exercise/physical-activity-guidelines-children-and-young-people/

NHS. (2019c, October, 8). *Exercise.*https://www.nhs.uk/live-well/exercise/

NHS. (2019d, October, 8). *Physical activity guidelines for older adults.*

https://www.nhs.uk/live-well/exercise/physical-activity-guidelines-older-adults/

Pearse, C. (n.d.). *10 Benefits of Calisthenics Training: Calisthenics vs Weights.* Atemi-Sports.

https://www.atemi-sports.com/benefits-of-calisthenics/

Perry, M. (2020, October, 20). *7 primal movement patterns for full body strength.* Built Lean. https://www.builtlean.com/primal-movement-patterns/

Petre, A. (2020, August, 7). *9 natural sleep aids that are backed by science.* Healthline.

https://www.healthline.com/nutrition/sleep-aids

Piacquadia, A. (2018, February, 9). *Training buddies makes exercise so much easier.* Pexels.

https://www.pexels.com/photo/young-slender-female-athletes-giving-high-five-to-each-other-while-training-together-in-sports-club-3768722/

Porter, E. (2020, March, 17). *Should you start doing calisthenics to get in shape? (pros & cons).* The Trusty Spotter.

https://trustyspotter.com/blog/calisthenics-pros-cons/

Quinn, E. (2020, November, 8). *The principle of progression in weight training.* Very Well Fit. https://www.verywellfit.com/progression-definition-3120367

Ramchandani, P. (2020, April, 8). Covid-19: *We can ward off some of the negative impacts on children.* New Scientist.

https://www.newscientist.com/article/mg24532773-000-covid-19-we-can-ward-off-some-of-the-negative-impacts-on-children/

Rampton, J. (2016, August, 30). *The importance of food, sleep, and exercise and how it impacts your success.* Inc.

https://www.inc.com/john-rampton/the-importance-of-food-sleep-and-exercise-and-how-it-impacts-your-success.html

Red Delta Project. (n.d.). *Core chains.*

https://reddeltaproject.com/calisthenics/core-chains/

ResMed. (n.d.). *10 common types of sleep disorders and how to identify them.*https://www.resmed.com/in/en/consumer/blogs/types-of-sleep-disorders.html

Roam, A. (2015, May, 19). *Intro to movement patterns, and why they matter.* Roam Strong.

https://roamstrong.com/movement-patterns-intro/

Robertson, K. (2017, October, 6). *20 great reasons to exercise.* Get The Gloss.

https://www.getthegloss.com/article/the-top-30-reasons-to-exercise

Robles, A., & Robles, B. (2020, October, 6). *The complete list of calisthenic exercises [beginner to advanced].* White Coat Trainer.

https://whitecoattrainer.com/blog/bodyweight-training

Rogers, P. (2020, November, 2). *Pros and cons of split system training.* Very Well Fit.

https://www.verywellfit.com/split-system-training-purpose-and-routines-3498381

Schifferle, M. (2015, June, 23). *Calisthenics regressions for strength progress.* Progressive Calisthenics.

https://pccblog.dragondoor.com/calisthenics-regressions-for-strength-progress/

Schroeder, B. (2020, February, 26). *10 reasons why you should go to the gym (2020 update).* Muscle Armory.

https://www.musclearmory.com/reasons-to-go-to-the-gym/

See, C. (2020, March, 25). *The cost of healthy eating vs unhealthy eating.* Plutus Foundation. https://plutusfoundation.org/2020/healthy-eating-budget/

Shvets, A. (2020, August, 9). *Man stretching with some yoga poses.* Pexels.

https://www.pexels.com/photo/senior-man-in-orange-shirt-and-black-pants-doing-yoga-5067957/

Sleep Foundation. (2009, December). *Nutrition, exercise & sleep.*

https://www.sleepfoundation.org/articles/diet-exercise-and-sleep

Soud, P. (2014, January, 27). *Benefits of whole foods vs processed foods on your health.* Fitness By Patty.

http://www.fitnessbypatty.com/whole-foods-vs-processed-foods/

Suarez, W. (n.d.). *Pros and cons of calisthenics.* Willpower Personal Trainer.

http://willpowerpersonaltrainer.com/pros-and-cons-of-calisthenics/

Subiyanto, K. (2020, June, 24). *Man doing wall push-ups.* Pexels.

https://www.pexels.com/photo/photo-of-man-doing-wall-push-ups-4720311/

Suni, E. (2020, July, 30). *Healthy sleep tips.* Sleep Foundation.

https://www.sleepfoundation.org/articles/healthy-sleep-tips

Testa, M. (2018, November, 23). *When is a sports injury serious enough?* Intermountain Care.

https://intermountainhealthcare.org/blogs/topics/sports-medicine/2018/11/when-is-a-sports-injury-serious-enough/

The Editors of Encyclopaedia Britannica. (2020, March, 26). *Calisthenics: Definition, history, benefits, & facts.* Britannica.

https://www.britannica.com/sports/calisthenics

Thevendran, G. (2017, June, 21). *Fastest ways to heal a sports injury: A medical perspective.* Mount Elizabeth Hospital.

https://www.mountelizabeth.com.sg/healthplus/article/fastest-ways-to-heal-a-sports-injury-a-medical-perspective

Times of India. (2020, May, 7). *Gym workout vs. home workout: The good and the bad.* Times Of India.

https://timesofindia.indiatimes.com/life-style/health-fitness/fitness/gym-workout-vs-home-workout-the-good-and-the-bad/photostory/75579201.cms?picid=75586756

Trainfitness. (2008, February, 16). *What are the benefits of circuit training?* Train Fitness.

https://train.fitness/personal-trainer-blogs/what-are-the-benefits-of-circuit-training

Tucker, A., Lappe, M., & Winderl, A. M. (2020, January, 4). *20 arm exercises without weights you can do at home.* Self.

https://www.self.com/gallery/sexy-arms-no-equipment-slideshow

University of Arizona Health Sciences. (2018, June, 1). *Sleep loss linked to nighttime snacking, junk food cravings, obesity, diabetes.* Science Daily.

https://www.sciencedaily.com/releases/2018/06/180601171900.htm

Verbanas-Rutgers, P. (2019, April, 9).*These trendy, intense workouts increase injury risk.* Futurity.

https://www.futurity.org/high-intensity-interval-training-injuries-2031452-2/

Visser, B. (n.d.-a). *Grilled chicken salad, a perfectly balanced meal.* Burst.

https://burst.shopify.com/photos/salad-with-chicken?q=meat+and+vegetables

Visser, B. (n.d.-b). *Man doing chest dips.* Burst.

https://burst.shopify.com/photos/strong-man-works-out?q=exercise+dips

Walker, O. (2016, February, 5). *Basic movement patterns.* Science For Sport.

https://www.scienceforsport.com/basic-movement-patterns/

Webb, S. (2015, June, 21). *Well defined shoulder and forearms on a woman.* Unsplash.

https://unsplash.com/photos/0DyZE6aLD-8

WebMD. (2019, October, 28). *Benefits of calisthenic exercises.* Jump Start.

https://www.webmd.com/fitness-exercise/benefits-calisthenics#1

William, B. (2020, November, 2). *Benefits Of calisthenics: How weight-free exercising can help you lose weight.* Better Me.

https://betterme.world/articles/benefits-of-calisthenics/

Woodruff, D. (2003, March, 3). *Movement patterns.* Personal Training On The Net.

https://www.ptonthenet.com/articles/movement-patterns-1937

Yu-Yahiro, J. A. (1994). Electrolytes and their relationship to normal and abnormal muscle function. *Orthopaedic Nursing,* 13, 38–40.

https://doi.org/10.1097/00006416-199409000-00008

Zelman, K. M. (n.d.). *Food to fuel your workout.* Jump Start.

https://www.webmd.com/fitness-exercise/features/food-to-fuel-your-workout#1

Printed in Great Britain
by Amazon